In th[e] [...]
Association ✓ **W9-BZX-227**

with great appreciation
to Cathy Lee and Ron —

Beyond Forgetting

⁂ who helped us through

Perci / Persei

/

See page 92.

Literature and Medicine
Martin Kohn and Carol Donley, Editors

Beyond Forgetting

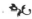

Poetry and Prose
about Alzheimer's Disease

Edited by Holly J. Hughes

Foreword by Tess Gallagher

The Kent State

University Press

KENT, OHIO

Contents

࿊

Foreword

TESS GALLAGHER

If someone newly returned from my future had told me in 1988 that I would spend the next third of my life caring for my mother, whose Alzheimer's seeped slowly, insidiously, like smoke over us for years, I would have been convinced they had the wrong person.

If this clairvoyant had also gone on to say I'd provide this care while fighting breast cancer, I again would have felt myself unable for such an assignment. And indeed there were times during the seventeen years I helped my mother, as congestive heart failure teamed up with the Alzheimer's to gradually put her through the many inflections of debilitation, that I wondered if I wasn't totally unfit to give what was needed. I had had no children, unlike my three siblings. Patience was not always my virtue. I loved solitude and had lived so as to preserve it to the benefit of my writing and teaching life.

I had initially returned home from Syracuse University to Port Angeles, Washington, where my mother still lived in 1989, after the death of my husband, Raymond Carver, in 1988. I had seen Ray through the ten months of lung cancer, and when he succumbed to the disease, I had ultimately resigned from my teaching in Syracuse and returned to the house we had purchased together in my birth town for the last of our life together.

We were widows together—my mother and I—gardening, reading some of the same books, consoling each other. I think she carried me emotionally during that time, as I wrote my way through the loss of Ray in the book of poems *Moon Crossing Bridge*. Later, when I began to work on a film with Robert Altman based on Ray's stories, she shared my excitement. Nonetheless, there were signs her health was giving way—groceries left in a trail at the side of the stairs going up to the kitchen, kettles boiled away, bills not paid, suspicions voiced that this or that person had taken one of her precious stained-glass lamps.

A different version of this essay, titled "Beyond Forgetting: Poetry About Alzheimer's," was given as a keynote address for "The Patient: An International Symposium" at Bucknell University on October 20–21, 2006.

She began to be unable to cook. I found myself carrying food to her; first twice a day, then three times a day. I began to stay until I saw her safely into bed late at night. As if I had held no other important purpose until then, I had come to her side. Doing so and all the subsequent choices I would make to support that initial choice are perhaps the most unacknowledged actions of my life, yet for that very reason, all the more sacred and precious to me.

As one of the few women loggers of the Northwest, my mother had worked in one of the most dangerous jobs in "the woods," as we called it, during the midfifties. She was a choker-setter who'd braved scrambling felled timber to place the thick cable around the log for yarding in to the landing. She'd worked with my father, a spar tree rigger and gypo logger. They'd had to make a living for five children, of whom I was the eldest.

My mother possessed physical daring, verbal wit, and what Ray called "an iron will." Add to this that at 91 she was still a beauty, capable of charming even the young doctor she saw the week before her death. She did not suffer fools. She could look to the center of a person and tell what they were made of. Stanley Kunitz, whose gardening and poetry she loved, held a special place in his heart for her, as she did for him.

At my father's death in 1982, Kunitz sent mother a Dawn Redwood to be planted next to her Bristlecone Pine, so their dialogue about which was the oldest tree in the world could continue at close range. The two gardeners maintained a flirtatious banter through news clippings they passed to me for delivery. Kunitz had visited mother's garden once in May and had seen her house-high rhododendrons in full bloom. But she had only my account of his Provincetown knoll, which was tiny by comparison with what she maintained alone—an acre and a half.

Marion Ettlinger, famous New York photographer of writers, who had photographed Ray so compellingly in his leather jacket, said her one regret when she'd come to take my own portrait for *Moon Crossing Bridge* was that she never got to photograph my mother. Mother had nicknamed her "the little pirate" because Marion dressed entirely in black, and when mother would think of her she'd ask out of the blue: "How's the little pirate?"

Mother connected with so many of my friends, though as her disease progressed, she could not remember their names a few seconds after they had left the room. After her death, I filled three manila envelopes with letters of condolence from writers, artists, and educators from all over the world. She'd managed to touch so many people with the dignity of her presence, her self-possessed way of sizing up things and speaking her mind, her no-nonsense, forthright assessment of anything said.

Her equanimity in the present moment had somehow been miraculously maintained as the Alzheimer's progressed, though many of the most important details of her life eventually slipped from her grasp. But because I managed to care for her myself in her own home for many years, and was able to take on outside help during my cancer treatment later on, I believe we became a kind of composite person. I supplied what she forgot, and she began to look to me to do so. On her side of the giving, she would interject stories from her childhood and mine, through which we came to know each other in new ways.

I recall especially her story of an incident in her childhood about a girl, with her mother, who had visited their farm in Missouri. She was told to take the girl out and show her around. While they were near the chicken coup, this girl said she was going into the house and tell her mother that Mother had threatened her with a hatchet. There was indeed a hatchet notched into the chopping block near the chicken coup. "I'll tell Mother you said you were going to kill me," the girl threatened with a smirk on her face. "What did you do?" I asked. "I just smiled back at her and didn't say a word. I knew my mother would believe me. And she did too. But can you imagine someone doing that to you? Well, I certainly never forgot her!"

As in the title of this collection of poems and prose by writers who also accompanied their loved ones through Alzheimer's, we did something unexpected, Mother and I: we moved beyond forgetting. Each day I bent my imagination, which had formerly been reserved for the classroom and the page, to discovering, for both of us, the best way to carry each hour, each day, each season.

We made wall hangings together, took holidays to the beach, and had afternoon matinees at my house where we watched old movies, especially those with dancing, which she loved. We peeled apples for applesauce and cut rhododendrons and iris for trips to decorate Ray's grave and those of my father and brother.

On one occasion in a cabin at the Pacific Ocean, mother got up at 5 A.M. the morning after we'd arrived and packed our bags. Somehow I managed to get us unpacked and reoriented so we could comb the beach for lucky stones and talk to strangers, which had been our pleasure in former times.

Living beyond forgetting, our given, was actually easier than one might think. It opened the universe of the moment and meant that in Mother's company, I had to be more alive than I had ever been. Javelins of insight and concentrated recognitions about the unadorned nature of that old cliché "being human" came to me daily in her company.

We were often silly together, as when her Boston terrier, Annie, jumped into the bath with her, and we decided to just go ahead and bathe her too, Mother calling for me to get the camera because she didn't want to forget it.

There were, of course, violent bursts of temper that would sometimes drive me out of the house, until after a few minutes, when she had forgotten, I could return. Rounds of the same story at close intervals made one deftly shift the subject. Meals became a ritual of refusals until I pleaded with the doctor to think of *something* to help her appetite. During her last weeks she actually enjoyed food, thanks to a medicine used to treat HIV, Megestrol.

Advocating for someone with Alzheimer's can be daunting for the caregiver, as when one realizes the spiritual responsibility it is to carry and accompany the loved one with Alzheimer's—a responsibility that is both satisfying and suffocating because there really is no choice at a certain level. One simply *must*. As I wrote of this in a poem, I seemed to be able to see the intricacy of what was required:

Can one soul consume
another? Or does asking violate
the notion: soul inviolable?
To ask is to wonder anew at the violence
of unseen forms.

Was it will over will?
Or did superior need bend us, one to
another? Does one who serves
hold the upper hand, having failed purposefully,
in the small ways, to mark and seal
parameters?
        (from "The Violence of Unseen Forms")

From stage to stage I kept insisting until I did manage to stimulate both doctors and caregivers toward the sense that even though her condition might be "hopeless" in the ultimate sense of what medicine could offer, there were still unexplored things we could do to make life better for her. By "better" I mean less confusing, more secure from her point of view, and more inclusive of her feelings and preferences, naturally with a view to protecting her safety too.

Perhaps my long practice of testing my poems' outcomes, their endings and assumptions, took a new form in addressing my mother's condition. Of the written arts, poetry is most responsive to the moment and so coincides with the condensed time frame of those with Alzheimer's—which oscillates between the distant past and the present moment.

Mother's long-term memory was always reeling in some strange fish from the past, even when she could not recall how her youngest son had died (in a violent car crash at age fifteen) or why another son lived in the same town but never spoke to her (the two having quarreled irrevocably). Perhaps she healed through the forgetfulness of Alzheimer's, for the tone in which she investigated these events was one of recovering something from a dream that I might also have had or that she had told me at one time.

During the last year of her life, she lived with me in a coil of oxygen tubes with the hum of converters cranking day and night. My sister and I marveled that all through her last year, she seemed actually to have improved in her ability to recall and connect things and to participate in conversations. When Alzheimer's is mixed with other diseases, it's often hard to tell why improvement occurs. Was it the oxygen? Congestive heart failure can rob the brain of the oxygen it needs to function well.

Another aspect of this regained ground was due to her having given over to my longtime wish that she get hearing aids. Again, I saw that the Alzheimer's had eroded a certain area of resistance. Taking the abeyance of temper as permission, I hurried to open up a new channel. She went through testing, got the hearing aids, and rejoined us and the world in an unexpected bonanza of alertness brought about by the simple act of being able to hear us.

Suddenly she heard birds again and rain on the skylights. She could tell exactly what someone was saying to her, instead of faking it and not responding appropriately. She spoke loquaciously on the telephone to her few remaining friends and to my sister who lived away. Some inner cohesiveness revived in her that final year.

I had taken mother into my home so the twenty-four-hour care could be woven more easily into my days while I underwent infusions of chemotherapy to which I commuted three hours each way weekly to Seattle. For seven months I lived with broken sleep, getting up several times a night with her. Finally, I added night-time caregivers to the one very able daytime caregiver. If I could say what I'd do differently, I'd get more help earlier. When one of the doctors told me it would normally take seven people to do what I was doing, it made a deep impression, but I was loathe to give over my sense of entrustment in the matter of Mother's care and postponed getting help for far too long for my good and Mother's.

As things became more demanding, both for me and for Mother, my grip loosened—a blessing for both of us. Mother was able to retell her stories afresh to the new caregivers. One was a wonderful listener, while another was an expansive and dramatic talker. Mother reserved her temper and stubbornness for a third caregiver, thus sparing us!

Just as the best poetry depends on an intensity of empathy, so the best caregiving requires an ability to feel with and for the one in need. The poetry I love most makes me *feel* the condition of another. Descartes predicated: "I *think,* therefore I am." Buddhism, as I approach it, exchanges this for: "I *feel,* therefore I am." Likewise with the poetry I love most—it makes me feel the condition of another. It often teaches me how to leap beyond the seemingly insoluble quandaries of situations. Poems carry us to the extremes of sorrow and unexpected joy, even as we search for meaning.

We tend to think those with Alzheimer's are the beneficiaries of our beneficence and mercies. But rather, in the wild unknowns they suffer, those with Alzheimer's draw from us heart's meat.

In my own case, I almost forgot I was fighting cancer, so focused was my caring for my mother. At the same time, she gave me something strong for which to live. I could be assured every day that I had much to give and a person I loved to whom to give it. Now, in her absence, the fullness of her presence shines anew. What for others was simply daily, for us took on the cast of the miraculous. How was it that even her sleep could inform my house with her exact presence? How could brushing her waist-length white hair, then braiding it as she had braided mine as a child, bring such a current of joy? One day we sat in sunshine on the back deck near the scent of lilies, as they unlocked her exclamation: "They smell so beautiful, they're shouting!"

When none of the medicines to stall off memory loss worked, the will to be with my mother in the best possible way could still be refreshed in how we went forward. As with so many things, attitude and the resolve not to cave in to the clichés of the disease, even its more ruthless manifestations, gave me something I could never have achieved any other way—an alchemy of spirit—by which the bond of mother-to-daughter could bring forth a birthing, moment to moment, in which memory was not queen. Rather, there was the murmur of unspeakable kindness passing as a gift with no giver—something that seemingly has little to do with identity or history. We let each other need each other, the blessing of that between two women who happened to be related.

"You're the mommy now," she said to me, with an impish smile one day. And so I was. And so I am. Meaning she had passed all she was into me, by the incalculable osmosis of her life conjoining with mine.

In the same way that the poetry and stories we find unforgettable pass into us and become an essential element of our bodily and spiritual knowledge, our encounters with Alzheimer's can lift us, even when they are most dire, precisely because they courageously enact under duress what moves us, makes us feel crushed or abandoned, tender and longing for things to be otherwise.

I do believe that those dealing with Alzheimer's may witness and help their loved ones more than survive. They may lead us beyond forgetting to the sites of meaning by which we continue to companion each other against seemingly relentless odds. Their knowledge within the community may move consciousness of the malady—loss of memory—past this identifying disqualification of disease. We may mistakenly think forgetting eclipses other human abilities when it most surely does not.

Preface

My mother died of Alzheimer's disease at dusk on the last day of April in 2001. At 75, she was still in good physical health—she had danced a polka just a few weeks before—so her death from this disease seemed all the more tragic. For my family, her illness had been a slow process of subtraction, as we lost her one brain cell, one synapse at a time. She had been an articulate, vivacious woman, and we had to watch her lose not just her memory but all that went with it— intelligence, judgment, dignity—all that we believe makes us conscious human beings. As the disease took away more and more of the person I had known as my mother, I had to look hard to see what was left. I tried to be with her where she was, but she drifted out of reach of reason, of our accepted ways of being in the world. How could I stay beside her in this journey? Words may have failed her, but I still had them. As with any grief that feels unspeakable, I turned to poetry.

Gradually, the practice of writing gave me entry into another world, a world larger than the small room where my mother's life ended. Writing poems made it possible to see that even in the darkest stretches, there were still moments of grace: her delight in seeing the scarlet flash of a cardinal at the feeder; rare glimmers of recognition in her blue eyes; funny conversations as the letters of her alphabet piled up. The losses may have been beyond imagining, but so were the unexpected gifts. Because she no longer had a past or future, she showed us how to live in the present.

Writing poems became a way to witness honestly while reminding me to dwell in the present alongside my mother. In our culture, we often talk about dementia only in the abstract, as a label, not in all its bittersweet concreteness. Many of us grew up hearing about relatives who, approaching the end of their lives, were "not quite there," "a little off," "touched." Now, because it is touching so many lives, Alzheimer's disease forces us to acknowledge it. I looked for other writing that might help me through this uncharted terrain. Each time I found a poem in which it was clear the writer also knew this territory I felt less alone. When I began to share the poems I'd written about my mother at readings, I came to realize how prevalent this disease is by the fact that a knot of people always gathered afterward to tell the story of their mother, father, husband, wife, sister, brother.

I began envisioning a collection of poems that might serve us all. I mentioned this idea to a few friends, who encouraged me to pursue it. I was, however, teaching full-time and enrolled in a low-residency MFA program, so set the project aside until I had more time. One day, at lunch outside on an unseasonably warm February day in Port Townsend, what was just an idea shifted decisively toward reality. Judith Kitchen suggested I contact Edward Hirsch, whose moving poems about his father were among those that had given me solace. That same week, Tess Gallagher, who was caring for her ninety-one-year-old mother with Alzheimer's, generously offered to write the foreword. Instead of a project I could do someday, this book became a project I would do now.

The response to my Internet call for submissions was immediately affirming; within days I received poems and essays from all over the United States, as well as India, France, Italy, and England. I was not prepared for this tidal wave. The hours between 11 p.m. and 1 a.m. became surreal, as I read poems that echoed my experience with my mother, essays so moving I was often in tears. When I wondered why I'd embarked on this project, I would read another letter, which ended with the words: *Thank you for doing this. It is much needed.*

As the deadline approached, e-mail messages stacked up in my in-box, manila envelopes piled high on my desk: poems and essays from husbands, wives, lovers, sons, daughters, sisters, brothers; poetry and prose from hospice workers, psychiatrists, doctors, nurses. Some wrote about caring for those with Alzheimer's disease, some had the disease; some experienced it, some imagined it. In painful, haunting detail each told of a journey, an experience that became more universal with each person's telling. As I read each piece, I began to better define what I hoped this collection would be able to do: to illuminate all the facets of this disease. The aim was made clear when one writer inquired whether she should send poems about the hard times or the good times. *Both,* I responded. *We need both.*

By the time the deadline came at the end of July, we'd received close to five hundred submissions of poetry and prose. I assembled an editorial team to help make the difficult choices. As we sat in my backyard one hot August day passing stacks of poems and essays among us, it was difficult not to feel overwhelmed. We wanted to encompass the whole range of the experience, to hear from as many voices as possible. We wanted to include writing not just of published poets, but of the people who know this disease intimately, the caregivers who have made it their calling. In the end, we chose pieces that portrayed the full spectrum: anger, frustration, despair, humor, tenderness, compassion. Because I was so often moved by the specific details in the cover letters, details that might help those who were caregivers, I asked the writers to provide a few sentences as context for the reader.

After the editorial team had made its choices, I retreated to Sky House on the Straits of Juan de Fuca to see how all the pieces might fit together. To the steady beat of waves against a rocky shore, I began to assemble the manuscript, finally able to see more clearly the many themes rippling through it. While the voices are strong, distinct, and each person's experience singular, I could see how the poems connected with each other and, I hope, with the reader's. I chose to group the poems and prose in thematic sections in an effort to make it more useful, and also allow the many haunting images to surface, sometimes next to each other, sometimes later, like an undercurrent.

In her essay, "Poetry and Uncertainty," Jane Hirshfield writes of the role of poetry in allowing us to enter into the unknown: "Poetry comes into being as a response to a kind of fracture of knowing and sureness: from not understanding, yet still meeting what arrives." The writers in this collection have done just that, meeting what arrives with courage and tenderness. Hirshfield also suggests how poetry might provide solace: "In entering the imaginative, metaphoric, or narrative expression of another, even if it is the expression of pain, longing or fear, you find yourself less lonely, accompanied in this life." This sentiment is echoed by Susan Ludvigson in the first section of her moving poem "Where We Have Come":

> To discover them
> is to link with the unbroken
> griefs we name and rename . . .
> to see loss
> black on white
> is to be comforted
> a moment
> in the early hours,
> not left alone.

In speaking with tenderness, these poems and essays remind us what we already know. As Linda Alexander writes in "Your True Life":

> Those who knew
> you when your mind
>
> tangled with a thousand
> worries whisper behind
> you, regret this stillness.

Yet here is your true life:
the bright, unruffled water,
a sudden lift of wings.

In speaking with honesty, these writers enable us to see not just the tragedy of Alzheimer's disease, but its odd dignity, its unlikely beauty. As David Mason writes in "The Inland Sea":

Their dignity another universe
might honor more than we do, seeing souls
where we see bodies falling into death. . . .
Their beauty terrifies us, so we think
it like no beauty we have ever known

and leave them for the ordinary shore.

I hope that the poems and prose in this collection affirm what Hirshfield proposes: "That anxiety, grief and the fear of chaos can be turned into beauty, meaning, and the irrefutable pleasure they bring, is no small part of the mystery of what art does." Through this transformative power, and in their honest, compassionate portrayals, may the voices collected here illumine the darkness of this passage and help us see, as one writer so eloquently put it, "the unlikely light that shines deep within it."

Acknowledgments

This anthology is the result of many minds, hands and hearts over several years:

First, my deep gratitude to Tess Gallagher for her moving foreword, for her belief in this project, and for the inspiration of her work and life, and to Stan Sanvel Rubin and Judith Kitchen, directors of the Rainier Writing Workshop MFA program at Pacific Lutheran University, for their vision and good humor and for encouraging me to embark on this project.

My thanks to Carol Donley and Martin Kohn, editors of Kent State University Press's *Literature and Medicine* series for sending the manuscript onto KSUP with their blessing, and to Carol Schilling for the assist. At KSUP, I am ever grateful to Will Underwood, the director, Joanna Craig, former assistant director and editor-in-chief, and Mary D. Young, managing editor, for their commitment to this project and their patience with my questions.

A deep bow of gratitude to the writers included here for trusting me with their moving and inspiring poems and prose, and for their patience with the lengthy editorial process. Thanks as well to all who submitted work; I wish I could have included it all.

I'd like to acknowledge the following colleagues and friends who stepped into the breach to help read all 500 submissions—Lela Hilton, Sarah Zale, and Marcia Woodard—and to my writing sisters, Patricia Nerison, Susan Sutherland-Hanson, and Barbara Brooking, for their careful reading, constructive feedback, and ongoing encouragement.

Thanks are also due to my colleagues in the English department at Edmonds Community College and to my dean for granting me leave to complete the anthology.

Former student Megan MacClellan and neighbor Myrna Keliher proved to be whizzes at Excel spreadsheets and exhibited great skill and patience for mundane tasks like stuffing envelopes and entering data, even though they are clearly capable of more creative work.

Three cheers to the first graduating class of the Rainier Writing Workshop for providing a lively writing community and, especially to Katie Holmes and

Kathleen Flenniken, who each provided valuable advice on this project when I needed it.

Words aren't adequate to thank my dear friend Cynthia Neubecker, whose belief in me and this project sustained me, even over many miles, and my partner, John Pierce, for his editorial expertise, surpassed only by his unflagging emotional support.

Finally, my love and gratitude to my sisters and their partners: Honore Hughes and Julie Gram, Missy Hughes and Robert Harris, and Stacy Hughes and Neal Anderson for walking this hard path together; to my father, Sidney Osborne Hughes for caring for our mother at home with patience and compassion longer than seemed humanly possible; and especially to my mother, Colleen Lindsay Hughes, whose bright spirit shone through even the darkness of Alzheimer's disease.

Beyond Forgetting

Alzheimer's

named for the doctor: Alois,
dead since 1915. In January 2002,
they link lesions on living brain
to the malady Herr Doctor mapped out
95 long years ago. Which could

mean diagnosing the living
positively: clear markers, no
doubt. No waiting for
the autopsy which means

the patient's a corpse
with a brain
some have likened
to Swiss cheese.

Just like the textbook slides
of that first postmortem.
That first, living,
patient got lost

in her own living room,
in her kitchen, in the sleeves
of her favorite dress. Bewildered,
she buried the china. Panicky,

she hid the knives. Cried
they were trying

to kill her. Screamed
when the voices were bad.

At last, her grown
woman's body, hugging
its knees to its chest, gave
itself up. Dead at 55,

emptied out, nothing
but flesh. It's this
vanishing act that we
call by his name.

Every day, less
and then less.

—*Mary Zeppa*

I.

Everything Framed
Against the Dark

❧

The Photographer's Father

JUDITH H. MONTGOMERY

waits beneath this maple risen
    in its late liquid cling of sun:
        October torch, leaves flaming

out of their bones, slope of shadow
    layered down the limbs, burnish laid
        against the dark thrust of trunk.

Beyond, the llamas' pasture plays
    one last green reckless hand
        against the stop and snap of winter.

A low sun picks out pod and thistle,
    burns its last waxed threads of wick,
        candling for the camera

the maple's winged branches,
    turning leaves as they forget their sap,
        crooked joints where storm or swing

bent things out of shape. Deep
    beneath this brilliant canopy,
        washed almost wholly in the dark,

her father rests, thick arms propped
    across the split-rail fence, one boot heavy
        on the lowest rain-grayed rung.

His hair alone blooms
    incandescent, lit above
        the bodyknot of shadows,

shoulder's bunch, collapsing
    fist of years. One knobbed hand
        stretches past the fence, the dim barrier.

His fingers—his gaze—
    stroke the muzzle of a llama
        young enough still to know its name.

The shutter stops. Look,
    this picture: everything
        framed against the dark.

"The Photographer's Father" responded to a close friend's photograph of her father in fall. In the afterlight of diagnosis, the season, the gesture, the brilliance of flame before it is extinguished, and his gentle touch crossing "that dim barrier" seemed to capture his present and his future, as well as her intuitive understanding of both.

Another Country

CANDACE PEARSON

Before she fully woke, beneath a cloud
of sheets that scuffled across her skin,
she was certain today would be different,
the clocks had already spun back on themselves
and she could slip between one second and the next
undetected. But sometime in the night

nouns had disappeared and when she tried
to say *clock,* it came out: *thing that goes round.*
She heard a whistle outside the window
and *bird* became *the thing that makes noise.*
There—*noise* was one of them, still breathing,
and she looked *for the thing that writes*

to capture the few remaining ones, searching
bedside table under dusty puzzle and book,
but the object had escaped with the word,
the way footprints succumb to the wind
or students who once cleaned her chalkboards
rubbed so hard no trace remained,

all for the sake of a gold star.
She had thought nouns might be the last
to go, naming carried that much weight.
No doubt surprised to find she had crossed over
to another country, one with no road signs, towns
without title, maps merely lines and elevations,

and she would need to make her way with verbs:
see, know, forget. Soon she would reach
the place where she could eat and drink. Relieved

of the responsibility of nouns, she felt
almost buoyant, unanchored as a thing
that flies—a *kite*—which has lost its child.

Language—our ability to connect with words—is crucial to me as a writer. I hadn't thought much about what it would be like to lose that ability until I witnessed it in my mother. Suddenly, her sentences had holes. I tried to honor that loss in this poem.

Across, Down

BRUCE BERGER

The daily paper's clotted wall of words
Confusing fact with fact, cause and effect
With yesterday's fact, no longer held intact
Unless it was tucked in half and creased in thirds,
Crossword on top. Braced on a crossed knee,
Stocks, cartoons, obits mere depth to write on,
Its chronic hints—stock pun, transparent clue,
Blackbird and *sloth* and *fescue* and *ossuary*
No longer necessary to look up,
Skewed definitions easily seen through—
Still held for words whose touch with life was gone,
Still peopled the empty squares, still played their tricks
Of intersection, weaving on his lap
A quilt of language purified of sense,
Irreducible as music or mathematics.
Head bent, mind still, bifocals glittering,
Surveying his princely grid of filled-in blanks,
My father took his verbal stance against
The nameless separation of everything.

I was struck that my father maintained his massive vocabulary and his touch with the wordplay of crossword puzzles long after he had lost his participation in daily life. I wrote "Across, Down" as a tribute to his talents that survived intact.

Elegy for an Amputation

RACHEL DACUS

They are disappearing like his toes:
first to leave is an *auberge* in Brittany,
then fishing the Sea of Cortez goes.
We start each telephone call with a litany
of events: *Remember, Dad?* Narrative salves
memory. We try to stitch it onto the stump
it fell from. Each visit our history's halved.
Conversation dwindles to plaints, grumps
and blame—*who put that bottle there?* His veins
narrow, synapses thin. Thoughts scatter,
drift and yet his brushwork remains
till another amputation—do fingers matter?—
when *now-you-see-him-now-you-don't* Dad
vanishes, leaving inch by inch and mad.

Old age is a hard country. My father, who has Alzheimer's, also developed a vascular condition that resulted in the amputation of all his right-foot toes. After several surgeries, the pain medication further scrambled his awareness. Between the two conditions, he was disappearing by inches. Losing someone to Alzheimer's is like small amputations: memories go away bit by bit.

Rushing to Return

ALICE DERRY

flotilla from OF, flote; ON, floti; OE, flota, ships

Leaves. Rain. Current. Fish.
Not Dad.
He's slow and breathless
as we gain the footbridge over the Dungeness.
He can still identify a few trees
and feel wild gusts in the air of fall.

When we left the house he worried
some of us were lost.
"Following," I'd reassured him, "in another car."
That's when he fastened on *flotilla*.

"Do you know where flotilla comes from?"
he asks now. "No," I say, thinking, maybe
it does come from Spanish, the Philippines,
where his fleet took days of shelling in World War II.
Sometimes he can still remember.

"From the Portland Rose Festival,"
he brings out, delighted. Is he drifting
back to the farm boy, breathless
as the parade's ponderous fleet steered through?

"By adhesion," he adds. I laugh,
but that's what Dad's lost—connection.

Of course, even then, say fifteen years ago,
when I gave him my first book of poems,
he wouldn't have thought of Whitman

as soon as he said adhesion—
word as *cover, blind.*

Dad was proud but asked,
"What about something substantial next time?"

Today works itself steadily toward rain.
Yesterday, cottonwoods against sky, gold on blue,
October caught me in the drama
between these trees, like wrought and burnished treasure,
and the end, which Dad too can feel in the air.

After the war he was a high school coach.
Taping up knees or ankles with adhesive
filled dinner talk, comradery of the simple win or lose.

Halfway across the bridge, we stop
for Dad to get breath. I want to see fish
rushing against the current, see what urgent
single-minded mission looks like.

"You can't see those fish in water," my husband says,
as if that's the point, water's great enabling miracle,
the peculiar sticky adhesion of its molecules,
here a kind of protective screen.

And when we lose the thicket words have woven
around us all our lives, as Dad has,
do we step free, onto this riverscape's
wide empty stretches of gravel, the record
of the channels it's tried and abandoned?

Dad's happiest if I stay right with him,
hold his arm, adhesion,
a steady attachment, grace of the middle ground—
what we never achieved,
locked most of our years in a fierce embrace,
despising what the other stood for.

Quit expecting so much.
Like what I do.
Hug me for me.
And I wonder what his list was.

The cottonwoods' tall autumn candles consume themselves,
giving off an incense, pungent, aseptic.
They aren't dying. Spring will sweep
the exhilarating fuzz of green across the valley.

Dad's granddaughters, ten years apart, have made a game:
who can catch the leaves spiraling down on the wind?
Seems easy, but they're elusive.

Each time he says a word like *adhesion* or *flotilla,*
Dad asks, "That's a word, isn't it?"
They're leaving him, one by one, and as he says them to me,
I write them down on slips of paper and hold them
to steep in my pocket,
thinking how they shimmer between us,
turning on their stems.

As dementia took its course, my dad began to lose his words. I tried to be true to
the ones he had left by using them in poems. When Dad said the word adhesion,
I immediately thought of Whitman using a kind of cover word, Adhesiveness,
for the relationship between men, as opposed to Amativeness, *which he used to*
describe heterosexual relationships.

The Tired Builder

BRIAN DALDORPH

He isn't getting the words right.
He knows it, keeps reaching
into his dark word-hoard
and brings up only apple cores,
fish bones and cool stones.
There *is* a word, he knows it,
for what he wants to say, but he's in a room full
of dictionaries and doesn't know where to start.
He'd give his right leg to have his mind back.
He's got cathedrals there
under construction,
but his stone masons can't remember
how to hold their chisels.
The window designers can only imagine plain glass.

The poem is written about a close friend of mine, a writer. He has a vast store of words, but he struggles now to find even some common words. I sense his great frustration, and his sadness.

Filler

LORENE DELANY-ULLMAN

Lovely, dear, lovely, he'd say, but he wouldn't say this, he would say, *I can't remember, it's you know, it's just gone. Justin, no, Christian.* And I'd pretend I can't remember, and I'd say oh, I forget things too. Yes, I do, really. *Lovely, dear, lovely.* Are you going? *Going where?* Mother says you can paint the kitchen white (she wants red accents, tea towels and canisters) even if you're going. I don't want you to go, *to go.* (In the background I hear the train, the train running its tracks, running its tracks.) He works in the garage, a mechanical pencil and index card in his pocket. With a sure hand, he writes and writes so he won't forget. (The train lays its horn across the tracks.) He falls asleep in his yellow recliner, the TV roaring. A tumbler of wine, another, and another on the table. *Stemmed glasses break,* he says. You're not going, I say. *Lovely, dear, lovely.* His desk was black with a smooth, shiny top and trim stacks of papers along its sides. He repaired watches there. He had a black lamp. Sometimes there was dust.

Much of this prose poem is a literal yet almost surreal depiction of a conversation I had with my father. This past year my brothers and I have struggled both with coping with our father's undiagnosed symptoms of Alzheimer's and with our mother's denial of his illness.

Erosion

DREW MYRON

Who knows how
the mind files memory?

Missing pieces, your
history, this life, lies
three states to the south—

lost rusted cars, bindweed
decay in the sun

wild geese fight winds
that rattle shingles, shake doors

your vacant eyes sort
through weeds, neglect

memory somersaults
lands against antelope
bones blanched in desert heat—

futile to search for data:
the face of a son, the hand of the wife,
price of wheat, words,
any words to rise, rescue us

from this wait,
this long silent loss.

*A silent question circled each visit with Bart Myron, my 94-year-old grandfather:
How does the mind file memory? In the days leading to his death, it seemed to me
that memory had the horrible power to both compose and erase a life, the critical
ingredients trapped forever inside.*

She Falls for It Over & Over

JOSEPH GREEN

Memory says, *Guess again:*
Which hand? Then switches
whatever it's holding.

It scrambles her recipes,
teaspoon & tablespoon,
pinch & cup,

steals salt from the shaker,
leaves sugar in its place,
an April fool waiting for her to taste

the clam chowder she would have made
if memory hadn't done something
with the clams.

When she thinks of the joke about
how we could have made an omelet
if only we had eggs,

it slips away, then pops
back up for her to tell again,
and she falls for it over & over:

We could have made clam chowder
if we only had scrambled clams.
If only she had a cup

of something that would stay
with its name, like flour,
like salt she could pinch & throw

over her shoulder for luck—but no.
Days from now the clams will turn up
stinking in a cupboard & the milk will

ripen overnight in the microwave
while memory says, *Guess again,*
guess again: Which hand?

My mother-in-law tells and retells scraps of old jokes and popular verse—"The
Little Man Who Wasn't There" or "I Eat My Peas with Honey"—but she can't
remember what happened less than an hour ago. My great fear is that I'll have
terrific recall but only for television commercials of the early 1960s: "Two! Two!
Two mints in one!"

Again, the Gnome and I Catch Dawn

SEAN NEVIN

A house is on fire
somewhere in the mind,
someone is trying to escape
someone is holding the other back.
　—MICHAEL BURKARD

Daylight opens across the lawn like disease
this morning, like fire traveling the rafters,

and the gnome and I are listening
to the brutal crescendo of woodworms
spit and sizzle with steam. They hiss
the hiss of the still alive, of the molted
blue claw left spattering in the grease pan,
and they set each riddled plank wailing
like a madman on the piccolo.

What if this is how it happens, how we lose
the stories of ourselves? Our porous bones,
like the timbers they are, already collapsing
into themselves. The burning eaves, ready
to buckle from the sudden lightness of it all.

What if this is my life, on fire,
the lit fuse of ganglia and synapse
sparking away like the gilded flecks of ash
that flare then vanish in the plume?

What if my life is the neighbor's howling dog
who has snapped its chain and gone begging
from yard to yard to be taken inside?

This poem is part of a series that looks at the phenomenon of sundowning, wandering, and garden gnomes. I wanted to explore the idea of the self and the multiple stations of consciousness that are revealed through Alzheimer's. Burkard's beautiful and disturbing image of one "self" trapped in its own disarticulating mind by another "self" was the seed for this poem.

Ineradicable

JUDITH BARRINGTON

Sigmund Gundle 1915–1996

He'll never forget their names: daughter
granddaughter, sister, late wife.
He'll always know where he parked the car
and what he went to the store for in the first place.

The President's name, today's date, his favorite
brand of coffee—all etched
like the names of the dead in a granite wall,
alphabetical. Memory's like that, isn't it?—

dark gray wall, file cabinet, a great room
with newspapers piled in rows by date and place
all of them recording news of a life
from gossip column to missile attack to the daily puzzle.

Or, of course, it's a computer: cerebral megabytes
swallow the story chapter by chapter
until the hard drive crashes . . .
What he thought could never be lost, *is* lost:

names escape through paneless windows,
streets sprout unexpected turns
and faces float away from their old histories.
He turns his wheelchair to block the corridor;

nurses beg him to move but he waves them away
shouting in German. So much is erased
but this he'll remember and remember:
the camp; the guards; yellow star; dead mother.

I wrote "Ineradicable" a few years after my partner's father, Sigmund Gundle, died of Alzheimer's. Toward the end of his life, when he couldn't remember the immediate past, his mind seemed often to dwell in the 1940s when he escaped from Nazi Germany after being arrested twice as Jew.

Blue Sonnet

RYAN G. VAN CLEAVE

Upriver, a swarm of flies. It's Spring. A deer
nimble across water, tragic how graceful.
Here in the quickening of nature, the life-span
of a man is best examined with tweezers
and magnifying glass. My father once said
Life may be a book, but with so many pages,
skip to the best parts. But the chapters he loves
are preface to me, *antes de* himself, even.

The placebo of names is not enough.
I want permanence, the rigid inscription
of DNA and sinew, the angelic
slow curve of hipbone. The bullnecked truths I want
are asleep somewhere, in a book perhaps,
a long-lost language, a casket rusted shut.

I was working on a sonnet sequence about my father's interest in genealogy when
"Blue Sonnet" emerged. It encapsulates a lifetime of awkwardness and also sug-
gests the fallibility of memory. The poem still disturbs me, which lets me know
it's a good one.

Five Minutes of Silence

ARLENE ANG

By midday the sheets lose their crisp mask.
His feet shuffle in sleep; this is not the first time
he goes missing: the lake froze one winter,
swans dripped away like Dalí watches,
Khartoum became synonym for ice, or else
apples someone stashed under the porch.

Is it easier to forget than to remember?
The pine in the garden sways, snow appears
like distant faces, the calendar has stopped
at June. We used to go fishing; there was
a trout that slipped through the net,
we had cold champagne in the boat.

Now Chianti in the cellar gathers cobwebs:
a process of aging. The red straw sinks
in his glass; he rarely complains of thirst.
An album lies discarded on the floor:
the past comes in unfamiliar snapshots
like a string of Buddhist prayer beads.

Alzheimer's disease is frightening because it happens without the person real-
izing it. And sometimes I feel that slipping into such forgetfulness can be as easy
as falling asleep.

Your True Life

LINDA ALEXANDER

You lost track of things.
Burnt the toast, forgot
to pay the phone bill.

One day you could not
decide the way home.
Someone took you

by the hand and led you.
Now everything is made
simple, all answered

by a smile or a nod.
In the late afternoon,
you watch ducks gather,

spread over the shining
lake. Those who knew
you when your mind

tangled with a thousand
worries whisper behind
you, regret this stillness.

Yet here is your true life:
the bright unruffled water,
a sudden lift of wings.

It is a challenge for a poet to understand a life without speech; harder still to
watch a man of words, like my father, journalist Holmes Alexander, fall into such

deep silence. Yet the simple, shining peace of sitting with him, as he gave up the daily struggle the rest of us are so immersed in, became for me a beautiful kind of meditation. So even now, after his death, when I sit mutely observing the small movements of the natural world, momentarily I can remember what matters.

II.
Azure Dissolve

Les Nuages

ELLEN KIRVIN DUDIS

Day after day she marvels at the clouds.
In the faded azure chair, in the shade
of an overburdened peach tree bowed
almost to the ground, she watches, half cloud
herself, the towering cumuloparade

and says the clouds are closer to you here
than in the city where she lived before
. . . or in the mountains? . . . She isn't sure—
her memory's only furniture
this azure chair, and all the fading years

beyond recall. One morning, tears blossom
out of the blue, she takes me by the arm:
*Have you my parents' address? . . . or . . . so awesome
a blank!* I show her the dates in the album,
Papa, Nana. *They've been gone a long time, Mom.*

She likes to tell us that the mackerel sky
means rain, as one who studies heaven's tea
leaves with a fortuneteller's eye—
names momentarily personify
the vagueness. A lifetime hangs identity

on mares' tails. Summer blazes on. My son leans
further and further into the *Moon-*
light Sonata, a mermaid figurine
flows from my daughter's hands and I pick beans,
hoarding the love and the guilt. What woman

with children of her own wants to mother
her mother? Still, when the thunderheads rear
each afternoon, I marvel with her,
glad for the wonder that slows her azure
dissolve. She's right. The clouds are closer to us here.

During her six-year decline to death from Alzheimer's, my mother was my respon-
sibility. She lived with us for more than a year, until we could no longer handle her
frequent panic attacks and found a wonderful nursing home with an Alzheimer's
facility. My experience as a caregiver found me wanting. My mother's memory loss
became my loss too: the frustration of dealing with her inability to think became
a burden, which obliterated my remembrances of her.

From *In Memory of Her Memory*

JIM NATAL

for Marjorie Bien Natal

IV
The horse that is my mother's memory
has run away. It hasn't gone far;
we can see it standing on the hill beside
our property, a silhouette at twilight.
I don't know who feeds or curries it now,
or if it has gone completely feral.
Sometimes the horse will come close, stand
just out of rope's reach. She calls to it,
then whispers of their past together.
The horse nickers and snorts softly
when she mentions Philadelphia or Chicago.
Its long neck extends and the horse shakes
its head when she talks about my father,
how she misses him, how people still
stop her on the street or in the grocery store
to tell her they miss him, too.
The horse doesn't seem to mind
that she repeats herself so often. No one
recalls when the horse got out
or who left the stable door open,
but perhaps the horse will return on its own
and we'll find it early one morning in its stall
munching hay and burnished oats.
We'll stroke the velvet blaze on its forehead,
reach into our back pockets
for those special carrots it loves.
And, if we're lucky, the horse
will linger for a while, maybe

lead us to the place where it last saw
my mother's missing hearing,
which also slipped away silently
while we were all asleep.

Poetry allowed me a way to try to deal with my mother's Alzheimer's—the despair, confusion, and frustration I experienced caring for the same physical person I had known all my life and trying to cope with the fact that that person wasn't there anymore. The "crown" of poems "In Memory of Her Memory" (from which this selection is taken) was begun while my mother was still alive and chronicles her descent and eventual death. It approaches the subject from many metaphoric angles, reflecting my attempts to explain to myself, and in essence to her, what was happening.

She Wipes Out Time

TESS GALLAGHER

like shaking horseflies from her white mane.
She would like to mail a postcard to
the place she was born. Not just to anyone,
but to the postmaster. *When I stopped to*
see him he'd gone out into his fields.
He had forty acres, she says. *I didn't*
go looking for him. I gaze across America, across
death to the postmaster, walking
his Missouri fields—wide sweep of farmland,
walnut groves, rivers and once-inhabited Indian caves
gouged into hillsides I explored
as a child by horseback.

A thousand acres, my mother says, restoring
them to herself and bequeathing them
to her children. *Your grandfather has a thousand acres*
That sentence, still a kingdom, though I know it never
belonged to anyone. The land gone,
but the words of it sustaining,
as if those acres—the vibratory memory
of them—were somehow currency to feeling able
for an expanse of loss. But who needs
a thousand acres? Better to have the thought
without the bother, to walk the mind under walnut trees
on the slope behind a barn long since
fallen away—as the mind falls away—the roots
exposed so the dry tendrils of small bushes
that cling bird-footed to air
remind us that air itself is a soil
apparitional to desire.

I too want to go back. Do go,
through the long stride of her wish
to make this sign of remembrance: a postcard
to the postmaster. In my mother's memory
of home, on which I lean, the postmaster still walks
his forty acres, though I know he is
long dead. Is it cruel to tell her
and obliterate that switchback
her yearning makes to resurrect him—who now
represents a place she can't quite reach
in her mind, except through the hyphenated corridor
of his perpetual looming up
as one broken promise?
I said I'd stop and see him . . . calm disappointment
in her voice. Why blot even false hope
to certify a useless truth? Any god
would let this postmaster have his saunter
in the mind-works of another. I say
nothing, let him live, beckoning to us both
across time, death and any upstart moment
that chooses her.

I am attracted to this new fold in time
by which a postmaster escapes death through having
gone for a walk. But, still the selfish steward
of this wild night-train of moon-blasted recognition,
I want her with me. "Mother," I ask, "when
did you last see him?" Her voice has the lilt
of truth. Memory's strange accordion crumples expertly
under the tail of the monkey: *Oh, a couple years ago.*
Mother, it's twenty years since you were back.
Then, making her arrow sing: *How time flies!*

By custodial violence I yank her to my template,
offer the card she wanted to send.
She forgets what it was for, uses it all day
as a page marker in her handbook
on African violets. Later she
reads deliciously aloud: *Water them
from the top and you'll rot the crown. Always*

let them take what they need
from the bottom—her reprimand steely
with innocence, so I suspect language itself
has flown defensively from the page into her
mouth with the audacity of particulate, unquenchable
matter that is, at any moment, fully able
to restore girlish laughter
to the high veranda, the postmaster's hand
closing vast distances
to my father's courtship letters,
ten years handing them over to her—letters
from her lover, far away in the desperate burrowings
of the coal mines. And now depths darker.
Twenty years toiling under us in the black ore of absence,
as the violets drink on their sills
from little bowls of the mind.

for Georgia Marie Morris Bond

My mother was a choker-setter in the woods outside Port Angeles, grew irises,
and told a good story. In her last years, she became me and I her; in that way, she
wiped out time.

Diminuendo

LARRY D. THOMAS

She first heard its onset
in the sudden, staccato
rhythm of her speech,
in the gradual diminishing
of brilliant memory

from chord to arpeggio.
Though largely confined
to the minimalist composition
of her nursing home room,
she still insists that the aide

help her daily with a black gown
and wrap her hair in a bun.
Positioned on her bench
with the straight-backed posture
she assumed as a concert pianist,

she sits at her only window
and watches the diminuendo of light
from afternoon to evening,
evening to dusk and dusk
to the endlessly repeated

étude of the night,
each of her long,
slender fingers
swaying like the winding down
needle of a metronome.

It's often said that people are what they do. "Diminuendo" is loosely based on the life of a friend's great aunt who, in the final stages of the disease, clung tenaciously to what still remained of the trappings of her art, even after she could no longer recognize the members of her immediate family.

My Uncle Chauncey drove my Aunt Eleanor

LEN ROBERTS

over two hundred miles every day because
she had Alzheimer's, couldn't remember
where she was, where she had been, and
had to see the elephants in the zoo again,
stop in to see her friend Rose
for the third day in a row. When
they left the house he had his teeth
clenched deep in his jaw, she
was smiling, sixteen again, bowing
to swoop up the tall-stemmed tulips,
oooing and aaahing as she looked into
the yellow and red, ripping the petals
off in puffs of circus colors just
before she skipped the rest of the way
down the walk. Sometimes she'd called
him Pete or William, or some other
man's name, and hold his hand a way
she had never held his hand, and
Chauncey would get jealous although
he was sixty-two and knew her mind
was riddled with time like the rotten
oak log in his back yard the carpenter
ants had eaten their way through. Holding
the car door for her to slide in, he'd shout,
Who's Bill, and who in hell are Merrill
and Ray, What in hell have you
been doing all these years? but she'd
just bend over to ask in that low, sweet voice
that had so recently come back, if he would
please peel out the way he used to, leave smoldering
tracks by the yellow curb in front of their house.

When I was a young boy, I used to visit my Uncle Chauncey and Aunt Eleanor in their home in Massachusetts. They were both very staid (and, dare I say, boring?) until, forgive me, she got Alzheimer's. At that point, she did very interesting things, some of which are described in the poem. As a child, I had no idea of the horror of this ailment, so I just delighted in her antics.

Everyday Cookies

CAROLYN A. DAHL

Glory's come: a woman of questions
who's losing all her answers. *Where are they,*
Sara? I've come to buy my Everyday Cookies.
Glory drops uninvited into a kitchen chair,
crosses her dried-bacon arms
on an old flat-ironed chest, and smirks
because she's remembered Sara's
home-baked rule that some cookies are
good enough for every day,
others meant for company alone,
with nuts, rice crispies, oatmeal,
chocolate, flour, butter, and salt.

Fixing a stare on Sara's plate of sliced salami,
Glory pushes a fork into the red flesh,
picks out the round chunks of pepper,
rolls them like BBs across the tablecloth.
Do you remember my Billy, Sara?
Died the day before our 55th wedding
anniversary. Do I have some, Sara?
Somewhere? Children? I've lost their names.
She counts the black pepper grains
into the bowl of a stainless steel spoon,
dropping the numbers like the names
of the children she can't remember.

What do I owe you for a tin of
your Everyday Cookies, Sara?
She opens her black casket purse
and pulls out a twenty-dollar bill,
uses it to scratch at her stiff white hair,

a green butterfly poking chicken feathers.
The bill bends, then falls, is sucked
under the table by the heavy breathing dog.

Then Glory's gone.
One hundred pounds of old woman
leaving with five pounds of
Everyday Cookies under her arm.
She guns the motor of Billy's Pontiac
and hangs a wrinkled self on the wheel.
All four windows open to August's fading light,
hair whiplashed by window wind,
she drives fast and furious,
white pearls chattering
at her neck like false teeth,
powdered face growing bright
in the rising dashboard light.
She's determined to outrun forgetfulness
and make it home without a stop.

This is a poem of admiration for a family friend who refused to surrender a ritual to the growing mind-blanks of her disease. Never knowing when she left home if she'd remember why, or how to return, she risked it all to buy cookies. I like to think she left us a message: to eat our everydays like sweet cookies until the tin rings empty.

Losing Solomon

SEAN NEVIN

We estimate a man by how much he remembers.
—RALPH WALDO EMERSON

Things seem to take on a sudden shimmer
before vanishing: the polished black loafers
he wore yesterday, the reason for climbing
the stairs, even the names of his own children

are swallowed like spent stars against the dark
vault of memory. Today the toaster gives up
its silver purpose in his hands, becomes a radio,
an old Philco blaring a ball game from the '40s
with Jackie Robinson squaring up to the plate.

For now, it's simple; he thinks he is young again,
maybe nineteen, alone in a kitchen. He is staring
through his own reflection in the luster and hoping
against hope that Robinson will clear the bases
with a ball knocked so far over the stadium wall
it becomes a pigeon winging up into the brilliance.

And perhaps, in one last act of alchemy,
as Jackie sails around third, he will transform
everything, even the strange and forgotten face
glaring back from the chrome, into something
familiar, something Solomon could know as his own.

"Losing Solomon" examines the many small losses, the daily subtractions and distortions of self, memory, and family suffered with dementia. It is not necessarily about, but lovingly dedicated to, my grandfather, Stephen "Snuffy" Kopec, a lifelong baseball fan. As I was writing the poem, it was his face I imagined in the toaster.

Verbal Charms

MELANIE MARTIN

Nana has been disappearing,
　　　　　　hands and nails and hair.
Each time I see her she's missing more,
　　　　　　　　another limb or tendon.
Her fingers are twisted twigs of arthritis
and her skin doesn't smell like White Linen.

*

She is not her *arroz con pollo, chilies con queso.*
No Christmas stockings hanging from the mantle,
　　　　　　　　no lemon or almond magdalenas.

Only a tiny Christmas tree with something on top.
　　　　　　　A teeny-tiny lady, she tells me over the
phone.

*

Her brain, a tangle of altered proteins
clumped inside cells I cannot see.

What I do see are her lips moving,
a word her mouth is forming.

She clings to my arm,
says, *Be careful. Watch out
for those people.*

*

She has been hiding things all day:
silver tin of molasses cookies stashed
below the nightstand,
                    cordless phone under the mattress,
money—easily 300 bills—
                    slipped between pillow cases.

                    *

Mom and I search her bedroom,
find a restaurant sandwich
wrapped in napkins. White toast, burnt and buttered,
so tough it could be a weapon.
                    Who knows how long it's been here, I say,
carrying the paper bags like a baby in my arms.

We leave red ribbons she has tied around lamps and picture frames.
A porcelain angel, one wing chipped,
                    watches over a photo of her daughter.

But even today she will turn to one of us, ask
Where is my daughter?
                    as if quizzing us.

                    *

Each time I see her she's missing more.
Her mouth, soft. Her hair, flat and greasy.

Her mind is slipping away, something I cannot catch.

She is a jellyfish.   She is a seal.

                    *

What was Nana thinking as she buckled a watch
on each wrist set to different times, hours apart?

Her past and present slide together like skates over ice.

One moment my grandfather is her husband,
then he is her father.

*

When I was eight, Lisa Wilson and I bet the neighborhood boys
we could stop gutter water with a wall of grass and twigs.
The boys swung high fives when the water broke our dam.

*

There is no water to break her dam.

*

I remove each watch
and set the hands to time
                even if time doesn't matter.

*"Verbal Charms" was inspired by my great-aunt, Nana, who had Alzheimer's.
The poem presents the struggle loved ones endure when everything familiar about
someone begins to disappear due to Alzheimer's.*

Finding Mother

SCOTT PETERSON

I found my mother
the other day, hiding
inside a desk drawer,
way in the back, behind
an old telephone book, next
to some loose change.

She was inside
an old pocketbook,
the one she hasn't used
in ten years, since
she began to wander, and
we took her keys away.

Just flip it open and
you'll see her, plain as day.
Pictures of sons and
husband, her two grandchildren,
neatly arrayed on top.
Then insurance and credit cards,
each tucked away in their own pockets,.
The driver's license, of course,
perfectly placed for easy display.
An old grocery list, some
appointment cards, all
square corners and right angles.

There she is,
all of her,
before she disappeared
and became something else.

One day I found my mother's pocketbook. Everything my mother was before she started down the slippery slope of Alzheimer's disease was in that pocketbook—loving mother, competent and organized to the extreme, on top of everything. Writing this poem brought all those things back to the surface—and that was a good thing.

Continuum

MARTHA MODENA VERTREACE-DOODY

By now I know your tricks by heart.
  You make me promise
not to watch you sleep midafternoon,
  your mouth falling open,
unraveling a skein of words. You will
  give the nursing home
one more week, you say, which means
  seven of something—minutes,
days, months. By your bed, a card
  of names and numbers
in large print, the daughter you call
  when the people
only you can see crowd the corners
  of your room;
real sons who will not disappear
  when you take your yellow pills.
I think of photos
  I have seen—

an artist's rendering of time:
  in a glass jar half-full of water,
a man coils, pressing white palms
  against the sides,
his black hair caught waving like sea grass.
  Naked, he lends color
as the camera finds what light there is,
  finds windows reflecting
glass on glass, tall windows like stained glass
  darkening a side chapel
at Candlemas. In another jar, more water,
  the artist's father, knees to his chest,

soles flat against the wall. I know now
   where you go
when you leave me, your mind
   trapped in space you touch
but cannot see: the alignment
   of eight planets and the Moon,

a child's connect-the-dots map
   to a mind set loose,
the surety of a black hole at the core
   of the Milky Way
where light breaks into nothing,
   returns to the dark stone
of matter. At home I try to draw your face
   but only manage
a creased paper bag, a crumpled page
   of foolscap,
a robe left hanging over a chair.

Several years ago I had the privilege of caring for the mother of someone I loved. Bess had Alzheimer's. As a poet, I felt drawn to record her struggle to let go as well as our struggle to hold on.

White Lilacs
Three Haiku and a Tanka

ANDREW RIUTTA

white lilacs
on a damp windowsill—
mother in diapers

autumn wind—
mother stares
where I cannot see

drift of pollen—
mother's journey
to another room

she's lost everything
that once retained the sunlight;
and yet . . .
her occasional glance
out the kitchen window

I humbly dedicate these poems to my friend Paul, who shared with me the pain of a son whose mother was becoming, more and more, less of what he remembered her to be.

At the Easel with Alzheimer's

RACHEL DACUS

My father is painting in the basement: blue,
green, yellow. The cinder block's wall white-
wash is tanned with dust and the ocean view
obscured by a flapping sheet of vinyl. It fights

the wind. He says he's inspired to blue. My call
comes to the studio phone. His greeting: *I can place
you. You're the pharmacist, right?* The pall
on his memory has not dimmed his bad taste

in jokes or how at the easel he's always affable
over the scribble of boar's bristle, the give
of canvas to brush. I skip over laughable
lapses, as when he asks me where I live

and then pretends he was kidding. Name-
dropping, his mind grows patches, nicks
and spores like the salt on his aluminum
windows that will eventually make them stick.

Painting down there, his panes always closed,
the air is warm and dry, not a hint of the sea.
What are you working on, now? His nose
nearly on the canvas, he can only say,

It's getting better, going somewhere. It's green,
blue and not as grim as it sounds. A brain
grows lacy and colors squirm like the skeins
of her yarns above the washing machine.
Don't fight the wind, I tell him. Be a net.
Catch the world by letting it slip the knots.

In my family, I watch the deterioration of my father. It's heartbreaking to see a rocket scientist lose the ability to use a computer, but it's also fascinating to see a lifelong painter sustain the connection with his past through the medium of art. My father is happiest these days at his easel, and what he has lost in intellect seems to be somewhat added back in an uncharacteristic peacefulness. The disease both gives and takes for all of us.

III.
My Mind Is a
Cold Oven

My Mind Is a Cold Oven

LANA HECHTMAN AYERS

i.
Alzheimer's Warning Signs:

Asks the same question repeatedly.
What day is it today?

Trouble performing familiar tasks, like preparing a meal.
How can this meat loaf be raw after an hour?

Forgets simple words or forgets what certain objects are called.
Have you seen my . . . those metal things that open doors?

Gets lost in own neighborhood and does not know how to get home.
Was that traffic light always there?

Has trouble figuring out a bill.
Five and Seven is . . . carry the two.

Repeatedly forgets where things were left or puts things in inappropriate
places.
How did my watch get in the freezer?

Becomes very passive, requires prompting to become involved.
No. No thanks, really.

ii.
On the five-minute ride home,
street names do-si-do
and I am lost,
swinging left, left, left,
before the neighborhood rights itself

and I am back two-stepping
up to my front door.

iii.
This watch face hides time from me
as my doctor's appointment
soups its way into abyss.

iv.
Neurologist says *dementia,*
but trained in math,
I hear dimension, dimensions,
impossible topologies of *n*-space
so complex and vast
they are terrained with Klein bottles,
trains on Mobius track
that never get where they're going.

v.
The oven's cold.
No supper.
I'm losing weight
without trying.
Who knew dieting
could be this easy?

*In 2002, I began having some frightening symptoms as mentioned in the poem.
Channeling the fear of what was happening into my writing helped me to cope.*

Early Alzheimer's

SHERYL L. NELMS

Emma set her
kitchen on
fire

because

she forgot
she was cooking

but the water

gushing through
the ceiling

for the bath

she forgot
she was taking

put it
out

I make a living as an insurance adjuster. This poem came from a claim that I had at work. It was a true story. The value of writing is ongoing.

Hot Flashes

ANDRENA ZAWINSKI

Aunt Mary always had hot flashes
that made her cry at weddings, at wakes,
as soon as her foot crossed the threshold.

At her skirt, the moment her hand squeezed
mine and our heart lines pressed close, my own
face flushed crimson with tears.
Aunt Mary cried when cats crossed her path,
at ladders too near doors: bad luck, bad luck,
she cried.

Summers at picnics, she tore at her blouse
in the heat, blazed: hot flashes, hot flashes.
She cried all the way
in the car ride back from the fortune teller
in Ohio who said, it's a spell—it's a curse.
She cried at the doctor's, big with a change-of-life
baby, bad nerves, high-strung, a flair for
the dramatic that ran in the family, but jumpy
as if her own shadow could be stepped
upon, pulled off, forever lost.

Aunt Mary still cries, mixing up
this face with that name the same
as always, but doesn't understand the new word
for it: Alzheimer's. Aunt Mary, who can spring
to her feet on all the quirky little steps
she remembers of the Charleston, waving
trophies in each hand, rattles walls
with gibberish now, explosive as nebulae
rising from mill furnaces she once stoked.

And I, I cry, bawl, blubber, have a knack
for the boohoo, too. I cry, hot, in the middle
of winter just watching the moon ride low
like a locket against the flushed breast
of night; and when a spark of star catches
my eye, I see: in me her blood runs red.

*This poetic sketch of my Aunt Mary presents a superstitious and nervous woman
wearing the curse of many women misdiagnosed by the health care industry or
by way of cultural myths. It acknowledges our link not only as niece and aunt but
as women. She died shortly after being diagnosed with Alzheimer's.*

Opera

GARY THOMPSON

Hours after the botched conversation, I'm kicking leaves on
my way to the car. It's dusk and streetlamps flicker on, one
after another, down the unfamiliar block—a synapse I can see
and follow like a path back to the known.

I see now that when Michael mentioned *Madame Butterfly,* the
sophisticated nub of my mind false-connected to *The Mikado.*
But stranger, the part of me that makes pictures, the side I trust
and love, sat me down in the audience of *South Pacific* and
wouldn't let me leave. My mother sat beside me, wearing her
Easter suit and green hat. Her perfume warmed the theater for me.
When she hummed "Bloody Mary," a song she and my father
listened to late at night after my bedtime, I thought I glimpsed
a flicker in the mysterious dark of adult love.

So when Michael said, "It's opera," and Arika and Steve agreed
gently, I stared dumbly into the disconnected air, unable to click
the lights back on up the aisle to the exit.

*My mother's Alzheimer's first became apparent around 1990, a time before there
was much public discussion, or available information, about the disease. Some early
research, however, indicated that there might be a genetic component, which caught
the attention of many sons and daughters of Alzheimer's victims, and certainly
colored the way we experienced our own moments of "botched" synapses.*

What's-Her-Name

BARRY SPACKS

My mother had Alzheimer's. Fearing combustion
she stacked on refrigerator shelves
her unread evening papers, laughed
to dazzle away forgetting the names
of relatives, friends, discarding at last
her own. I held her hand, unknown,
beside her bed as she babbled on.

With me if it's Alzh it's early, only
suddenly bridgeless synaptic gaps,
connections bombed away. I'll recall
in detail a book I read years before
or the layout of Barson's Drugs where I soda-
jerked at age fifteen, but not
some actor's or entertainer's name.

I can see this actress, her subtle beauty,
the delicate wit of her lifted brow.
She stretches her arms in her languorous way,
Ms. Nameless. So I work for recall:
remember some scandal-sheet lie about her,
the dress she wore presenting an Oscar . . .
maybe she'll whisper her name in my ear?

Names, names, they won't cross the border . . . !
I'll spend the whole of a Sunday morning
seeking the mock news announcer on *Saturday
Night,* that tumble-down-clown who suddenly . . .
Cybil Sheppard! Cybil Sheppard!
My God, you can't imagine the comfort,
dear Cybil, simply to speak out your name.

Nearing 75, memory a bit shaky, I worry about the possibility of approaching Alzh. My mother had the disease before it achieved its present name; "premature senility" they called it in her case. Should be easy for anyone aging to share the glee of the sudden return of a sought, lost name.

They

DAVE PARSONS

for Harry Dazey

Now that we know that Harry has Alzheimer's
we catch ourselves wondering out loud

about our own memories, searching
for that small void in our understanding

of time's continuum. This cruel wound
that delicately as some evil surgeon unseals

the mute gray bindings that hold
ineffably the inventory of a life

stuns us again and again with horrific wonder,
leaving us with facial expressions, not unlike his

as he turns his bent spade, again and again,
like some blind farmer through

the rough weed-filled furrows
of recollection and recognition.

At the Garden Café, Ruth stately still,
rotely asks him in that wifely way:

Would you like tea or coffee, Harry?
Harry, do you want tea . . . or coffee?

. . . then the realization . . . *oh . . . oh, give him tea.*
An acquaintance happens by the table,

and Ruth graciously, dutifully introduces her
to Harry, who, as always, smiles affably

and responds, *I am not really here,*
you know. Later, I accompany him

to the men's room, where he becomes confused
and begins to wash his hands before entering

·the small dark stall with its endless
roll of blank white sheets of paper.

Standing before the sink, he stares
with what appears to be rapt erudition into the mirror
and whispers in that familiar, gentle fatherly tone,
He wants to come back you know; he wants to come back

and they—they won't let him.

"They" is for my late father-in-law, Harry Dazey, who was on that awful precipice:
clinging to his still conscious world, but finding mostly those insidious "blank white
pages" when the incident that was the catalyst to the poem occurred. As I have
always said, Harry composed the poem; I just wrote it down for him.

IV.
Across the
Border

Across the Border

TESS GALLAGHER

for Greg

Into early morning we circle
the problem of his mother's dementia,
her cries of *help me! help me!*
ricocheting against the stars
even from the balcony of this posh hotel
across the Canadian border
where he and his family are like refugees
of some secret war-torn country
within the country. I sit with him
the way a mountain sits with another
mountain, comparing weather,
the slippage of glaciers, the racket of
helicopters searching for lost
climbers, anything that spoils our
violet reveries with the night.

His hope-coffers are empty.
She doesn't know who he or anyone else
is. She thrashes wall to wall like
a trapped bird. No one wants to help
him take care of her—the waiting lists
at the facilities up to a year.
I need something, she tells him, *but
I can't tell you what it is.*

She hasn't slept for days.
The medicine that opens the sleep door
doesn't work on her. The anti-psychotics
don't tamp down the fear anymore.

She's like watching a lightning storm
over a lake, doubled and single-minded
at once. No comforting arms
for her. She won't be placated. She's
a force now, like wind or rip tide
uttering unanswerable edicts as it
dashes things to pieces. He dashes
each suggestion I make. Too late
for that. Or that.

Now we know why the old women
are lighting candles in the dark alcove
of the church, kindling a wavering city
of light, white candle burning next to white
candle. Maybe that's the trace hope leaves
when it's emptied out by crude events—reduced
to a sign, a silent cry made of light.

*Maybe those who have met the full unreasonableness endured when a loved one
suffers the effects of Alzheimer's are the best comforters of each other. This poem
recalls my staying up much of one night trying to console and help my friend,
whose mother is described in the poem. It did a world of good for the two of us to
just talk and listen. Often there is no way to make the situation less painful or to
change the outcome for our loved ones. The pain just has to be acknowledged and
even ritualized as in the ending of the poem.*

No Destination

PENNY HARTER

Having no destination, I am never lost.
—DOGEN

I.

"There are fifty people in here,"
my father tells me, "and some of them
walk round and round all day."

He carries questions in his pocket,
fingering the keys that used to mean
something, the coins that go nowhere
but his palm.

He has been trying to get home
from a voyage lasting ninety-four years.

What mast has he tied himself to?
What crew has plugged their ears
against his cries to be unbound
as he struggles to break free?

He would swim through rapids
toward voices that call out to him
at night, luring him somewhere,

anywhere, away from his body
breaking down, his mind
whose strings are snapping
one by one.

II.

Before the accident, my father
did not know his destination
would be an eighteen-wheeler
stopped at a red light, and we
did not know that Mother's life
would end so soon.

A few weeks afterward,
as we rode together on some errand,
my father's roughened fingers closed
around my hand as if he were drowning.

But I cannot save him from himself,
hauling him to safety on some shore
he'll know as home.

There is no map for that.

On a December evening, my father drove into the back of a stopped tractor-trailer.
After severe injuries and a valiant struggle, my mother died seven weeks later, and
I got legal guardianship, putting my father into an assisted living facility for some
months before his death. I felt such contradictory feelings, ranging from love to
extreme hurt and frustration. I had been teaching The Odyssey *during this time,*
so I used that imagery as an extended metaphor.

Odysseus, Mortal

RICHARD BEBAN

Afraid of his next step he clings to her
who mothered reluctantly, who sees

marriage end as it began, one last child
supplants her proud king. She waited vital

years for *this?*—to watch him lose his slow brawl
with memory, calling her Calypso

or Circe, deaf to her corrections.
At night he screams shipmates' names as he dreams

the one-eyed giant. She is sorry he
lashed himself to the mast, didn't succumb

to the sirens—wishes for him Hector's
sword had been true. He who risked the domain

of shades now a fading sallow shadow.
Imitating her work, he unravels

his life each night, waking to find weft threads
gone, absent skills to weave himself back to

Ithaca, back to her, back to himself.

"Odysseus, Mortal" stemmed from hearing about so many friends' parents going through this horrible descent. But it was triggered by watching the experience closer to home; seeing how the caregiver suffers so deeply as well—perhaps even more—when both have been so strong and so long coupled.

My Grandmother's Teeth

CHRIS TUSA

My grandmother's teeth stare at her
from a mason jar on the nightstand.

The radio turns itself on,
sunlight crawls through the window,

and she thinks she feels her bright blue eyes
rolling out her head.

She's certain her blood has turned to dirt,
that beetles haunt the dark hollow of her bones.

The clock on the kitchen wall is missing its big hand.
The potatoes in the sink are growing eyes.

She stares at my grandfather standing in the doorway,
his smile flickering like the side of an axe.

Outside, in the yard, a chicken hops
through the tall grass, looking for its head.

*I wrote the poem shortly after my grandmother was diagnosed with Alzheimer's.
My hope was to write a poem that used stark imagery to convey the horrors of
the disease.*

Accretion

PETER SEIDMAN

i. Angst—June 1988

My mother creeps into madness—
And I watch.

Once the dancer   never a person of the mind
She's become deaf to her world   and herself

A program of ever-repeating ever-decreasing

Ever-shortening subjects

Repeating
Ever more incessantly

Death bad restaurants long-ceased family feuds
Restaurants European anecdote her differences
With siblings . . .

Love breeds sufferance

Yet I succumb to fear
Yelling at deaf ears.

And what of my father?

Long suffering himself shuffling patriarch
Finally accepting winter-time

He reasons   he knows

He hears my mother's creep.

Damnable dilemma:

Sacrifice himself
Or put my mother on the stone.

ii. From a Dream—November 1996

Ungrounded
Graying about the gills
Dream's eye sought her out—

My Anima.

Finding her—
She invites me in
With gentle hands   long thin fingers

Velvet skin

These hands   the grounding and the gateway

To madness or awareness.

iii. A Thursday Kaddish—September 1997

The son asked to bear witness:

Your face is yours
Your cheek   cold   smooth
As when   at bedtime
I loved to touch it   velvet.

Now well on your way   migrating
Through fireworks and demons dancing

You are   and always were

A bird.

The sun shown Thursday
The sky sierra blue   deep and clear
A late summer breeze.

Above your pine-cloaked body
A leaf-shadowed tree. Within

A crow calls.

I smile   you are laughing

Crow Mother

Agent of beginnings and conclusions
Who wing   bob   shuffle

Not just forlornly stand

Chortling commentator to our chilling keen
You caw down to us

Don't grieve
Dance for me.

My mother's disease was never tragedy to me. She taught me that one always has a choice: to laugh or cry. As she crept into ever-worsening Alzheimer's (thus the poem's title), she never lost her joyful engagement with life. And so I laughed too, and with the laughter came clarity. "Accretion," written over several years, is my mom's description (with me as scrivener) of her tiptoeing journey into places unknowable except by those along for the ride with the likes of her.

From Missing Script

CARA SPINDLER

Four:
Paint a black hole on the floor

for when we start to forget, at the end
of our time. Don't cry, pet: if I remember
everything, I will live over, maybe
a little backwards, again, love.

that the patients will not cross
because infinite bottomless forever
lost like cows their eyes slide past

the seal on her chest she dressed it
for him and the calendar is now somewhere
down to their wedding day running

away tomorrow night his scratch
her window makes a gap the way a tooth
missing aches where a soul

has located itself on the floor in front
of her door through which enters
her grandson brushing past her to open the curtains

on the night's breeze the two wedding
dress sleeves chiffon billows they call
the nurse forgets to shut the window

she was planning to tonight or was it last
night if she waits he will climb in
late will he come through the door

will he come down the hall again the way
that he can step over the abyss the sucking trap
like it is nothing he is still tall

in front of all the exits she has seen him
step right over it he pauses at the holes
and checks it to save her
from wandering alone if only
mad fierce burning anger because he is late
from work and the morning's remainders

sitting here all day where has his soul
located itself in this world that he looks so young
who is that woman who follows

laughing mouth open crimson like a reminder
she bobbed her hair had had long beautiful hair
was it last week holds palm up to chin reassured

short and they say "his chair" and every
forgotten birthday comes to mind these days
when left alone for eclipses eons pass

as wide as the atlantic a train ride to
jersey where one day he promised
a vacation will take care you forever

the peonies a kiss but wasn't it her birthday
yesterday all these cards they can't help
and the calendar always wrong too many

occasions visitors a vacuum when they change
decorations but lights are always up like
christmas and all those touchstones gone

This poem is excerpted from a five-poem cycle entitled "Missing Script." My grand-mother dealt with Alzheimer's in the last two decades of her life, until 1992. The final place she lived was a long-term care facility specifically for patients suffering late-stage dementia. I do not remember it as a happy place; at the time, there was even less research about treating the disease.

V.

I Do

I Do

E. A. AXELBERG

True that this is what you signed on for
in such bodily earnest before the distractible
justice of the peace 64 runaway years ago—
another sleep-skimming vigil in the spool bed
(your one and only), on guard for any sound
or movement from the shadow beside you.

In the steely wash through the open windows,
you wonder what it would have been to say the words
in this era of gimcrack vows; to have cut and run
before it came to these long nights, long days
of thrown spoons, the fixation on *going home*
and the childhood stalwarts you keep him from.

For now, he sleeps gently, on some spar he'll let slip.
Hard by you, the old tabby breathes in his own
singular dreams of constancy; and you, you lie
in this invited light, recalling the kiss the J. P. forgot.

*Watching my mother care for my father over his years of dementia was a reminder
that love deals in surprises and will take us places we never expected. The poem came
from her experience and my imagining being in such a place of loving loyalty.*

Rev. Robert A. Young (1893–1977)

GARY YOUNG

Verily I say unto you, Whosoever
shall not receive the kingdom of
God as a little child, he shall
Not enter therein.
　　—MARK 10:15

Ill, shaken and hollowed out, he remained
the best of what he had been, the mad preacher
delivering sermons to the wall, entreating
the curtains to be wary of their pride.

This man once held me
spellbound from the pulpit, the only preacher
I could ever sit still for.
If age stole his vigor and withered him,
he avenged himself with good deeds
and better. If the world was lost, spirit
was everywhere waiting to bless and be blessed.

I still see him standing in the fog
of his failed senses, hands gesturing
to a phantom couple who have come
to be married by Dr. Young, here
in the corner of the bedroom.
Do you take this woman, he asks,
do you take this man? And I hear them
answer each in turn, *I do, I do, I do.*

My grandfather, a Methodist minister, died of Alzheimer's disease in 1977. He had always relished performing weddings, and in his dementia he would often perform ceremonies for couples only he could see. I always thought it was fitting that as he drifted further and further from the rest of us, his refuge was a place of union, a place of love.

The Married Man Keeping His Vows

MARY ZEPPA

In sickness, in health. In Alzheimer's.
59 years slipsliding away. Like my dream:
in your bed, on your knees swaying
over her, just as you

were about to begin. You had lifted
the hem of her nightgown by its blue
and delicate edge, when
befuddlement

dropped its cloud over you,
sucked you up into its folds.
On your knees, then, and whistling
for courage, till the hang of it flooded back in.

*My parents had been married almost 60 years when my father died. Theirs was
a love story. My father was a very married man. In his last three years, however,
my mother had essentially become his caregiver. This poem, a complete work of
fiction, literally came out of a dream.*

From The Alzheimer's Sonnets

RONALD PIES

Sonnet for a Missing Singer

The doctors say some pinkish sludge
is what does you in. Gobs of amyloid
and twisted strands that just won't budge
from the brain. Pretty soon, a void
of neurons hangs like some old
moth-eaten sweater, where once
a solid weave of bold
thought reigned. Yet the soul hunts
for clues among the mind's gray runes,
and now and then finds some Rosetta
Stone of memory—an old Sinatra tune
that brings back spirit, if not the letter.
Love, these cells that wink out one by one
are not the song of all that we've become.

This sonnet is one of four that seemed to spring out of nowhere. I think the words "The Alzheimer's Sonnets" actually generated the poems themselves. Somehow the juxtaposition of the eponym "Alzheimer" and the beautiful poetic term "sonnet" set off a strong emotional reaction in me. Of course, my experience as a psychiatrist must have prepared the emotional soil for this unexpected seed, as did my personal involvement with friends and family who have experienced declining memory in their later years.

Absences

ETHNA MCKIERNAN

Cell by cell my mother is leaving us.
No one can stop the memory leaking
from her body in such helpless cupfuls,
the way flecks of dead skin disappear
and scatter into air like loose dust gone wild
when brushed from sun-dried flesh.

The lost language in her eyes,
my face before hers like a question mark,
her vision blank with Haldol
or bright with terror,
a terrible incomprehension
stuttering through her body—
I hear the doctors say her brain
has atrophied a few degrees
beyond the CT scan of last year,
and I see a border of grey air
circling that unprotected, shrunken mass,
empty spaces wind could rattle through,
small animals could chatter in.

The howl at the door. Each day, every night.
Down the road, a gravesite beckoning.
My body like a fetus, curled in mute rage
on the floor near her bed. Selfish
as an infant, wondering who will know us now,
when we were children.

My mother, in all her Irish beauty,
singing suddenly at 3 A.M.:
The violets were scenting the woods, Maggie,

displaying their charms to the breeze,
when I first said I loved only you, Maggie,
and you said you loved only me.
My father, weeping.

During the years of my mother's Alzheimer's (1991–96), I wrote a sequence of poems
that I ended up titling "Alzheimer's Weather" after her death in 1996. None of the
poems was planned but arose purely from the moments and months she was sick,
and my own need to keep from drowning as I watched pieces of her leave each day.
"Absences" was the first poem I wrote about my mother's disease, in the year before
she went to a nursing home; "Potatoes" was written several years later.

Potatoes

ETHNA MCKIERNAN

Someone is weeping in the kitchen.
It is my father, crying quietly
as he peels the dinner potatoes.
He pierces their white hearts with a fork
and steam rises upward to his beard.
Below, hot tears salt the bowl.
The intimacy of the moment staggers,
as when I stumbled, once, as a child,
upon him cupping my mother's face
in broad, noon daylight as they entered
the deep, private zone of a kiss.
How could he have known, when he made
that vow fifty-seven years ago,
how suddenly and readily she'd leave him—
pork chops burnt, potatoes blackening
over gas—for that thin stranger
called Alzheimer, waltzing through
the kitchen door like a suitor
who has never lost a single lover's hand
he's played?

Nostalgia

STEPHEN MEAD

Dream within dream, this translucence almost
parallel, superimposing bubble heads pressed against
touches or the feeling that there's some squid spread
presence upon upon . . .

Wake up sleepy, you're
eighty-five & it's delirium, these lips in-
escapably bent over, colt at a brook, water under
the bridge . . . It was spring. We were walking. Clear
clean air, your laughter, contagious: axles doubled
out of mouths, spinning faces . . . Neither here nor
there because, later, slamming doors, I found your
fury humorous, though scared of, that word, the
divorce . . . Our hearts, sudden peg legs tottering
on a sea-sloshed deck, hardening reluctance, boxes . . .
I didn't know where the hell your old football
jersey was and & why should I, damn, care . . . hitting
my finger with the hammer hanging that wreath
the trash coughed up our fourth xmas . . . flirting
with the grocery clerk, eggnog woozy . . . "It wasn't
anything, Marsha!" . . . Of course, silly, seal-eyed
out of the tub . . . your nice climbing body I
rather preferred . . . where are you . . . the radiant
way of . . . squabbles, smooches . . . back a step . . .
back . . . we'll see . . . we'll . . .

Alright, I'm coming to. Stop prodding.
Not dead yet. Here is my face, fork.
Come bring my dinner

"Nostalgia" is a rather eccentric poem first written in the early '90s. I believe what first inspired me to write it was a meditation on the lives of my grandparents, an empathy that later came in handy when I worked in nursing homes and hospitals. One of the most important things to remember about the geriatric is the richness of their interior lives, that they are tapestries of experiences lived.

To My Father, Now on Liquids in the Tucson Nursing Home

JEFF WORLEY

Mother, whom you no longer know,
raises the cup of blended carrots to your mouth.
You open. And I want you to give out

with the latest joke you've heard or tell me why,
again this year—as we watch Sosa round third
and get nailed at the plate—the Cubs aren't worth

a goddamn. The orange liquid doesn't stay down.
Mother changes your bib. Friends tell me,
savor these moments; one day he'll be gone.

Now she spoons vanilla pudding into you.
Good, you say, and open again, waiting
for the cold spoon to settle with the sweetness
of what's left to you.

*In several of the poems I've written about my father's Alzheimer's and his death,
I've tried to explore and dramatize the role of his primary caregiver, my mother.
She's the hero of his Alzheimer's story, though her intense caring for him for so
long also took its toll on her.*

At the Alzheimer's Center

TIM MYERS

He's just dropped her off,
his wife of thirty-seven years.
For him, this is what mornings are now:
this gray midwinter heaviness of sky,
this thing he must keep doing.
Their conversations are oddly casual
but with a strange circularity:
"Here we are, Martha," he'll say flatly;
"Oh? What is it?" she'll ask.
Sometimes he answers with a quiet smile,
but even when grief lurches through him
he's always tender.
"The Center, honey. It's time to go to the Center."
If you saw him later, in the aisles at Wal-Mart
or watching TV in his reclining chair,
you wouldn't know:
just an old blue-collar guy like a million others,
ball cap, graying mustache, bit of a swag-belly.
Old wolf in the lean deeps of winter,
he fights an inextinguishable hunger
hour after snow-muffled solitary hour—
fights even now, as he pulls up to the hardware store,
not to glimpse in memory
the woman she was.

For seven years my university office was just down the hall from our campus Alzheimer's Center. Those seven years were an education for me, a "curriculum" of overheard conversations, random encounters in the hallway, glimpses through the Center's open doorway, and—as in this poem—observations I couldn't help but make in the parking lot. I learned a lot about darkness, but I also learned about the unlikely light that so often shines deep within it.

Carlos y Norma

MAUREEN OWENS

Near the end of life we stop getting dressed.

Like Carlos, we live in diapers and pajamas
it is unlikely he will ever step out again.
He yearns for underwear, his legs
floating inside silk boxers.
Norma does not know him—*ese hombre,*
que tu vez ahi, ni es la sombra de mi esposo—
and he is not even that, this
mere shadow of her husband.
She puts on earrings, necklace,
makeup with her pajamas,
carries her accessory case everywhere.
Yesterday, Carlos said, *estoy regresando,*
soy otra vez un bebe.
Maureen massages their birdy backs
through thin pajamas; Maruchy translates.
They are old these babies,
they have stopped getting dressed.

And we all lose ourselves, becoming babies again.

I wrote this poem while assisting my partner with the care of her parents. Norma has Alzheimer's; Carlos died in June 2005 at the age of 92, devoted and deeply in love with his wife of sixty-eight years.

Dementia

PERSIS KNOBBE

You're a queen, he says.
I'm a queen? I stop whipping the egg whites.
And, he says, AND (he nods wisely) you have money.
I'm a queen and I have money. I like the sound of that. I'm a rich queen.
Yes.
Nodding wisely, I tell myself: Now *that* is dementia.

After a long stint with Alzheimer's, my husband spent ten months in an assisted-living facility before he died in the spring of 2005. I am writing now about the before and after of placing him. I like to think that we did our time with a mix of humor and grace. (That is what I like to think.) In this poem, a man with Alzheimer's sees his power ebbing in the early years of the disease. He no longer calls the shots. He sees his wife in charge of everything. Now she is everything.

The Strains of Memory

JANE ALYNN

Most days, she sits in the wheelchair
where she's been since her fall,
broken femur that never healed.
Whatever she wanted for herself
when she married, the prospects
long abandoned, like the Beethoven
sonata that throbbed in her concert pianist
hands or love a body longed to know,
was carefully buried
and now pokes out like bones.

But today
she flashes an angelic smile;
her face gathers a blush like afterglow.
She smoothes her pink pleated skirt,
brushes thin hair, soft as ash,
trues her tiny frame in her chair
and spills the news, not able to hold it.
For the first time her body feels
alive—a new fluttering, touched
by a man, recently admitted,
whose kisses arouse lost desire.
She lets him into her bed at night,
when he wanders the hall,
and they lie in perfect harmony.
She has forgotten her past,
the husband who visits Mondays,
says *We're getting married*—
a sentence that fades to a tremulous silence
as she strains to remember this man's name.

I always imagined the onset of Alzheimer's would be morose, or worse, torment-
ing. How could the loss of one's mind not be? The wretchedness of forgetting? And
yet, visiting with my mother-in-law, I am amazed at her passion, courage, and
happiness. Listening to her, I hear the creak of a door opening.

How

GILBERT ALLEN

many years has it taken me
to realize you, Barbara,
are my best story?

I've given my life
to that lofty country where the truth
is no excuse, even
at that left, sinister margin
when every fact, face will leave us
nothing at all.

But from that almost-first
meeting, at a summer dive, at midnight,
when I honestly believed your sorority sister
with the bobbed hair and pantsuit
was your implausibly short, silent
boyfriend (till I happily
noticed, through a dozen daiquiris'
daze, his purse)

to when I picked you up
at your parents' house and remembered
seeing you at the Beach Boys concert
six months and three hundred miles
earlier, and told you where
you'd sat, and the color
and cut of your winter coat
though on that February evening
I'd never seen your face

to finally today, nearly thirty
years later, when your mother stumbles headstone-sober
into our bedroom at dawn and asks who
in the world you are
and speaking yourself through your sleep
you ask back *Who do you think I am*
and she happily decides
A good friend—

how
in hell or heaven
can I better that?

*Cecilia Szigeti died on Easter Sunday, 2002. During the final years of her life,
she suffered from both kidney cancer and Alzheimer's disease. I first saw her in
1972—on the day after I'd introduced myself to her daughter, Barbara, who I had
the good sense to marry in 1974.*

Spouse as Home

ESTHER ALTSHUL HELFGOTT

I didn't know he
was my *shul*
my language
my mother tongue
and prayer
the *zeyde* I lost,
and *bubbies*
I never had.
Or that he was my homeland.
And exile.
My nakedness.

I didn't know
when I met him
twenty-five years ago
that I had needed
a place to
dwell
in.
Or that knowing
turned less
into more
And more
into
less.

Oh,
where
shall I dwell
when he's
gone

Where
shall
I
when
he's

I was born and raised in Jewish Baltimore, where secular, religious, and leftist Jews lived side by side. I did not leave home to come to the Pacific Northwest until I was 29 years old, in 1970. When I met Abe, my husband, who had grown up on the religious end of the Jewish spectrum and was well-educated Jewishly, I saw someone who embodied aspects of a life I had left behind. Only when he became ill with Alzheimer's did I realize fully that when I lose him, I also lose a piece of yiddishkeit *and the neighborhood I grew up in.*

Nocturne

AILSA KENNEDY STEINERT

My words glance off your hard silence,
the tiny sips of your answers, your impenetrable
self. Listen. You are a French town,
lane by lane, hiding its gardens.

It's been so cold. A swallow darts
against the mirror of the stream.
In the field where I have run the dogs,
roses spill their hearts out.

My husband grew up in France, and, in past years, we have been in many French towns with their high walls and closed gardens. As his dementia increases, I have been struck by the similarity—all his riches are closed off and hidden. Now, we see only the outer surfaces.

VI.
What's Enough

Short-Term Memory Loss

MARK THALMAN

Mother, a Phi Beta Kappa,
who graduated second in her college class
and could have become a doctor or lawyer,
although women back then
were not encouraged
to do such things,
now cannot remember
where to find her glasses, keys, the car
left in a tow-away zone,
ice cream and hamburger thawing
in the trunk, golf clubs swimming
in milky blood.

She watches the same video of Lawrence Welk
three times in a month.
The toilet,
she forgets to flush.

Talking to me on the phone,
she will discuss only the weather,
and if I ask to talk to Father,
lays down the receiver
to look for him
and does not come back.

She knows she has trouble remembering
but can't recall why. When her husband
explains the word Alzheimer's,
she tells him, "If I go insane,
I'll commit suicide."

Sitting in her favorite chair,
she compulsively clutches
her thread-worn sweater,
a security blanket, while I
read her a story,
as she would to me,
before I could decipher
the words.

My mother's symptoms became noticeable when she was 53, and she was diag-
nosed with Alzheimer's two years later. Then she slowly declined for the next eight
years. Alzheimer's is usually thought of as an elderly person's disease, but this is
not always true.

My Mother Doesn't Know Me

LINDA ANNAS FERGUSON

To her, I'm the mild-mannered woman
who cooks her meals.
She is going to leave me
a tip when she finds her purse.

She sits for hours, eyebrow
cocked in a wrinkled study,
as if she can fathom
the distance between us,

saves pieces of thread
in a coffee can,
picked from her afghan all day
while both our lives unravel.

Thanksgiving, she put a hammer
in the oven at 400 degrees,
spent the rest of the day
on the back porch step,

wanting only to leave
this strange house,
silently wringing her hands
as if her body could not contain her.

"My Mother Doesn't Know Me" was inspired by my former mother-in-law, Rosalind
Knox Ferguson, now deceased, who had a brilliant mind. I often struggle with words
to try to convey loss and the uncertainties of life. When I walk down the stairs, her
empty chair meets me, listening.

Safe-Deposit Box

ELIZABETH FARRELL

In the box at the bank
there is nothing but dust.
Yellowed papers about a car
you have not driven for years.
Old tickets from a movie matinee.
Nothing there worth the price
of maintaining this safe-deposit box.

Every day you accuse me of stealing
piles of money you insist is there waiting
to be counted and used for your pleasure.
You rub my finger raw looking for the ring
you tell me I have taken from the box.

When I wipe the peaches from your chin,
and try and kiss your sour lips with love,
you do as you always do: shout loudly
that I am the one who has taken each precious gem
from the safe-deposit box, simply because
I have the key you can no longer hold.

*I wrote the poem to reflect the condition of Alzheimer's and how it betrays both
the afflicted and the caretaker.*

Ukiah Afternoon

ALLAN DOUGLASS COLEMAN

Small-town California courthouse, August:
I'm stuck in summer school again, this time
for repetition of a course I didn't fail,
relearning what I know too well: she's here
and yet she's gone. On the stand an expert
offers gifts of truth that no one would unwrap,
explaining massive insults to the brain,
dementia, and such. My brother breaks;
he has to leave the room, but I stay on.
It's not my time to cry. I'm here to watch
my mother sit and smile, look aimlessly
around, then catch my eye and wink. Inside
me a balloon fills drop by heavy drop
with grief, but meanwhile I blink back,
answering her call on the duty of blood—
thicker than water, thinner than tears.

My mother, Frances Allan Coleman, began exhibiting Alzheimer's symptoms in the mid-1980s, around age 70. The diagnosis became official in the early 1990s, during the course of an unnecessarily protracted and painful competency hearing before a small-town Mendocino County circuit court judge later removed from office. She died in November 2000.

Concerning Ice Cream on Mom's Side of the Family

ALLAN DOUGLASS COLEMAN

Her father Jim's my childhood
memory of love. Daytimes
in summer I would ride
the cowflop-crusted flatbed
of his truck or sit the cab,
his sawdust sweat combined
with turpentine into the finest
aftershave, as he'd go paint
a barn or build a porch or wrestle
a reluctant bull-calf
to the ground. Sometimes
he'd have me clean the henhouse,
heave some bales of hay.
Then we'd soap up, scrub off
in a fraternity of foam.

Evenings after dinner he and I'd
sit at the kitchen table, there
to play casino for an hour or so.
Her mother Emily would bring us
each a heaping dish of ice cream
homemade in a freezer tray:
the cream from cows I'd watched
him milk (I never did learn how),
mixed in with chocolate pudding
from a box. Dense, crystalline,
it fought the spoon and stayed
forever on the tongue, taught
patience to a young boy feeling
cherished, chafing at affection's
always steady pulse but oh so slow.

I didn't know that once
I was in bed and they'd closed
up the house, Grandma
would don her nightgown
and then wash her feet
on the announced assumption
that she'd die in sleep that very night
and didn't want the neighbors
finding her extremities unclean.

Years later, over ice cream
at my mother's place, I told her
I walked through my city
like a prince. It shocked her
that I felt so good: she blurted out
"Not like a prince!" to strip me
of my joy. It was a reflex action,
uncontrolled, unplanned, her way
of warding off the evil eye.

Her long-dead mother is alive
and ill in her. For ten years now
Mom's plotted her own end,
rehearsed the where and how of it:
pills, alcohol, a leap to the ravine
or slow submersion in the lower
pond. Then there's the when,
the advance notice given, ceaselessly
revised, like the horizon sometimes
near but always beyond reach:
on her next birthday, two years
hence, before the winter cold
sets in. She's a sly huckster, shilling
her own shuffling off the coil.

Most recently it was to be this fall,
once her grape arbor's harvest
had been pressed for wine. But she
misplaced those words. Into
that vacuum of forgetfulness

rushed other shards of memory,
dense, crystalline, and what popped out
was this: "I think that I will kill
myself when they've made ice cream
from the hens." I had to laugh, and you
can too; it doesn't bother me.
What else is there to do?

Time pivots on its heel, and suddenly
I'm back inside that farmhouse kitchen
forty years ago. Knowing what I didn't
know, I watch Granddaddy Jim
drink sunrise coffee, Grandma fry
an egg I gathered—hear their rooster
crow while, silent in the freezer,
dessert hardens for the evening
meal. In this dominion of slow melt
I'm only a pretender who'll renounce
the throne one day and vanish
from the hall. This prince
of ice cream is no prince at all.

What's Enough

CATHERINE WILEY

She calls to ask me where I am,
   as if I, too, were lost: the cordless
      phone goes missing once it leaves

her hand, the phone call, too, erased
   in minutes, her next call an hour
      later to demand what I have done

with the blue ceramic bowl
   bought at the Duchess County fair
      twelve years ago, the one with Queen

Anne's Lace imprinted on the sides.
   A dozen bowls fill boxes
      in my basement; I lie and say

I'll look for it and know next week
   the bowl will be replaced by a jug,
      a scarf, or no request at all,

just a sigh that sleep comes hard,
   she doesn't feel like eating, the staff
      can't cook, there's no taste left.

Not me, I say, not this way,
   this extended expiration,
      this diminishing (her own

mother square and solid, pearls
   tucked smartly in the wattles jiggling
      as she chewed, until the night

she simply died in bed). Now my
    mother plods the gaudy aisles
        of Kmart, propped by a cart, me

one step behind, extra diaper
    in her purse, admiring the stuff
        no longer with an eye to buy,

just glad to know, perhaps, it's all
    still there. Sometimes letting go
        takes years of tepid sloughing off,

lapses and forgettings chisel
    deftly toward some core, some bright
        bead that rolls just out of reach.

Of what use now my keen-honed skill
    at dodging her, frenzy paled
        to pettishness, edges blunted,

aim askance? She's shrunken to
    compliance, fear of breakage tempers
        every step, and each time I believe

this phone call is the one to set
    in motion my arrangements, I
        submit to her flimsy keeping on,

mottled houseplant sending out
    a stubborn bud or two in spring,
        each breath not yet worth counting.

"What's Enough" is a meditation on how much physical life counts as living, rather than surviving. Whenever I suspect that my mother's greatly circumscribed situation is less of a life than she deserves, than anyone deserves, I remind myself that none of us can know what is enough.

Fudgesicle

ROB HARDY

He can still make his scissors say "bread,"
paring away the word
from its picture in the weekly specials,
cutting holes to represent his hunger
for the thing itself, now that he's lost
his taste for naming.
He fills an envelope with pictures
to represent fulfillment—

a full loaf,
a gallon of milk—

and my mother does his shopping,
coming back as always with her arms full
of unspoken things.

He's lost weight, too—
as if the fat were in the words
he no longer uses, as if the extra pounds
were simply forgotten—
like the word for fudgesicle.

I remember him saying once, angry
when my siblings and I had eaten all the fudgesicles
without leaving the last one for him:
"You know how I love fudgesicles!"

I don't remember him
ever saying how much he loved me.
But now that he's lost the word
for "fudgesicle," I realize that what he really loves

was long ago
already beyond words.

A few years ago, my father was diagnosed with Progressive Supranuclear Palsy (PSP), a disease that shares many characteristics with and is often misdiagnosed as Alzheimer's. Research on PSP frequently adds to our understanding of Alzheimer's and vice versa. One of the shared symptoms of the two diseases is aphasia, the loss or impairment of the use of language.

The Strangers in Your Room

JOHN GREY

I could be the mailman for all you know.
What's this? No letters.
Or maybe I'm the baker, the one
who used to leave the newly cooked loaf
on the top step beside the milk bottles.
And no, I'm not the milkman either.
You surely don't believe that I'm the teacher,
the strict one I used to hear so much about.
Besides, she was a woman.
You do know the difference, don't you.
You'd rather, I'm sure, that I was an old fishing pal,
come to the door with creel and poles,
with bait enough to last a week,
and saying, "Come on Charlie, the trout are biting."
I'm anyone but me I figure.

You stare at me like I could be familiar,
but then you turn away.
I'm just one more flower in a vase, one more
photograph you shake your head at, one more
half-eaten cinnamon roll on a plate.
Or maybe I'm your father, the one
who didn't know you from a quilt pattern
in his last days.
You told me once how cruel that was.
So I'm cruelty.
Glad to know you. Glad you don't know me.

*This poem has been growing some years, cocooned in my experience with a particu-
lar uncle that I was close to but who gradually lost his memory, and it was almost
as if our relationship was drifting backward into an ultimate nothingness.*

Down and Around

JOHN DAVIS

I have been the Chinese proverb
If two men feed a horse it will stay thin
I have been law-abiding
and the laws I have abided by
from time to time I have broken
like the hard thoughts I have broken

across my forehead
from eastern daylight to pacific daylight
been sober with my mother
when we've lugged my father
carried his anger, his body
his Alzheimer's mind to a bathroom.

I have been the horse
I have been the hay and I have been
sickled, baled, unbaled
chewed up for fuel
slid down and around
a thousand-pound stomach
excreted into handsome green balls
fertilizing rose beds.

I have been the fertilizer
I have been the rose
so how about it, Sugar Lips?
In the spongy autumn twilight,
let's march inside this bar
and take whatever blessings
the beer gives us.

The simple task of helping an Alzheimer's patient to bed can take hours. My mother's internal resources seemed endless as we assisted her in caring for my father. "Down and Around" was written following such a session. By including various narratives and personas, it allowed me to highlight this struggle and to locate its place within our daily challenges and opportunities.

On July Nights I Stay with My Father

JAN HARRINGTON

Because he is vehement
and I am tired, I let him wear
his winter boots to bed. Their clasp
of his ankles calms him—an antidote,
I imagine, to the loose
helplessness of pajamas.

Later he sits up, shaking,
cries out: "Where are my shoes?
I need shoes."

"You're wearing your boots, Dad."

He stares at me, sees *stranger,*
not *daughter.* I am slight ballast
for his night terror.

"How did you find me?" he asks.
"Will we make it out alive? Whatever
happens, stay here."

He sleeps. I wait,
a sentry at the mouth
of the painted cave, watching
for morning's pale rim.

The progression of my father's illness led him, like a pilgrim, through time. In the early years I could accompany him by recognizing the people and landscapes. He spoke to his mother about crops; worried about six-year-old me out in a storm. Eventually he entered a world where he journeyed alone.

The Bath

HOLLY J. HUGHES

The tub fills inch by inch,
as I kneel beside it, trail my fingers
in the bright braid of water.
Mom perches on the toilet seat,
entranced by the ritual until
she realizes the bath's for her.
Oh no, she says, drawing her
three layers of shirts to her chest,
crossing her arms and legs.
Oh no, I couldn't, she repeats,
brow furrowing, that look I now
recognize like an approaching squall.
I abandon reason, the hygiene argument,
promise a Hershey's bar, if she will just,
please, take off her clothes. *Oh no,*
she repeats, her voice rising.
Meanwhile, the water is cooling.
I strip off my clothes, step into it,
let the warm water take me
completely, slipping down until
only my face shines up, a moon mask.
Mom stays with me, interested now
in this turn of events. I sit up.
Will you wash my back, Mom?
So much gone, but let this
still be there. She bends over
to dip the washcloth in the still
warm water, squeezes it,
lets it dribble down my back,
leans over to rub the butter pat
of soap, swiping each armpit,

then rinses off the suds with long
practiced strokes. I turn around
to thank her, catch her smiling,
lips pursed, humming,
still a mother with a daughter
whose back needs washing.

My mother was diagnosed with Alzheimer's disease in her early 70s. For the last year of her life, bathing her was a constant challenge. On this particular day, even though I didn't succeed, what was a contentious situation transformed into a moment of tenderness we both needed.

A Little Less Than the Angels

CLAIRE KEYES

My brother doesn't read books,
except for the Bible, his choice
even before his wife became his baby,
slumped in her wheelchair, rolling her tongue
around her gums as if searching for
missing teeth. And who is he
smoothing her hair, pressing a cup
of water to her lips? He points to tracks
he's rigged along the ceiling, the pulleys
he's attached so he can lift her from wheelchair
to toilet to bed, careful to tuck her knees,
her feet, checking her eyes for signs
of comfort or distress. Evenings,
he pedals his stationary bike and reads
the Psalms, reciting them over and over
to keep from falling asleep.
Because it's tiresome and lonely,
though he doesn't complain.

Weekdays, he escorts her to day care,
staying to play the banjo and sing tunes
for the old ladies who nod and tap their feet.
"Let me call you sweetheart," they sing along,
making eyes at him, loving him so much
they want to take him home.
My brother is a lover.

He presses fifty pounds on the shoulder machine
at the Y, bathes his wife three times a week
and needs his strength so she doesn't slip
from his arms. Then what would he do

to Praise the Lord, all He hath given,
all He hath taken away?

First comes my brother Richard, a remarkable human being, and his loving care of his wife Dorothy for the past eight years. Then comes a poem by Wislawa Szymborska, "In Praise of My Sister," which helped me see a way of writing about my brother without being maudlin.

Passing the Hat

M. J. IUPPA

for Louis A. Iuppa, M.D., at 90

My father, the good doctor, is patient,
sitting perfectly still in his chair; thin
arms crossed in his lap with five
of his favorite hats stacked on top
of his head.

We are moving back to the city,
closing the lake house for another winter.
My mother speaks to me in few words,
and I understand what steps need
to be taken.

We work at the same time but alone,
glancing out bedroom windows at the new
stretch of beach; the lake mirrored blue
as the sky without wind or cloud, believing
that we'll be back as we bundle summer
clothes in bedding and shut doors behind us.

I pass my father—once, twice, three times.
His pale blue eyes follow me; he smiles but
doesn't shake his hat heavy head.
He gives me "thumbs-up," reaches
to the top of his hats, and tosses me one.
In his effort, a chuckle catches
in his throat. He turns his face away
until it passes—
              This is the way it is.

Tentatively, I
place his cap on my head—he watches me
pull the brim down over my eyes, and asks,
Are you ready?

My father wasn't able to do the grunt work required in our family's moving from the lake house to the house in the woods. So, in humor, he put all five of his hats on top of his head, just like the man in Caps for Sale. *That was the last year my mother would move back to the house in the woods. My father's dementia increased with my mother's passing. So much of his present tense was tied to hers.*

Mamababy

JUDITH ARCANA

Mamababy, she's all small now
real thin and light
you can see her
bones and tendons greywhite
through her speckled skin

she's losing weight
a nice young doctor tells her to eat
she's not hungry but she tries
she wants to be good
she's frightened, sometimes she cries

she opens her shaking fingers and cries
I've got no strength in my hands
I've just got no strength in my hands
then she subsides into the big chair
real quiet, because she understands

she shuffles from room to room
like a footbound woman
Daddy does the laundry, cooking, cleaning
but she can still dress herself

she takes a long time
so he has to wait for her
like when the children were young
and she dressed them all first

oh, that was so long ago, she cries
so long, they're old now
the children are old

Rick and Julie have grey hair
and Teddy's bald

even then, though she doesn't remember this
even then she would be
handing a jar to one of the children
here baby, open this for me
you know I've just got no strength in my hands

This poem is rooted in the keenly felt effect on the rest of the family. An upsurge of memories among us—the younger, relatively healthy, folks—provided fiercely ironic commentary, and fostered frequent examination of family history and relationships in our conversations.

Pacific Sunset

ARTHUR GINSBERG

A rat's nest of tangles and plaques
chokes my mother's brain,
as she sits on Chesterman's Beach,
fiddling with her grey wig,
unaware of the egg-omelet stain
that batiks her blouse, and telltale
wet spot between her legs, oblivious
to the booming Pacific that stretches
before her befuddled eyes, the salmon-pink
sunset I have brought her to see.

There's our house, son,
she says, pointing to a cloud,
and, *Isn't Montreal beautiful?*
In the next breath, she berates me
for marrying a fat cow, then asks,
a moment later, if she has said
anything wrong. I cling for comfort
to the sough of beach wind through
stunted pines. *Reuben* (my father,
gone ten years), *I want to go home,*
now, she whines, a bewildered smirk
on her face. Sure, Ma, I reply, and I take
her arm, light as a bird bone,
steer her back to the cabin I have rented.

By candlelight, I spoon into her mouth
mammaliga, the corn gruel she loves
from Pietra Namsk in Romania,
where she grew up. What tenderness
I hold for this marred mind, how fine

to have known this palace of her spirit,
the template for mine. Lip smacking
speaks to a wordless content,
as she sundowns with the light,
leaves me holding
an empty bowl in the dark.

A few years before my mother passed away, when she was in a moderately advanced stage of Alzheimer's dementia, I invited her to come from Montreal, my birthplace, to Tofino, on the west coast of Vancouver Island. I rented a cottage on the beach, where we enjoyed sunsets together and I fed her her favorite food each evening. After she died, the bittersweet memory of this time expressed itself in this poem.

VII.
Lay Back the Darkness

Lay Back the Darkness

EDWARD HIRSCH

My father in the night shuffling from room to room
on an obscure mission through the hallway.

Help me, spirits, to penetrate his dream
and ease his restless passage.

Lay back the darkness for a salesman
who could charm everything but the shadows,

an immigrant who stands on the threshold
of a vast night

without his walker or his cane
and cannot remember what he meant to say,

though his right arm is raised, as if in prophecy,
while his left shakes uselessly in warning.

My father in the night shuffling from room to room
is no longer a father or a husband or a son,

but a boy standing on the edge of a forest
listening to the distant cry of wolves,

to wild dogs,
to primitive wingbeats shuddering in the treetops.

*This poem is a prayer. It is based on—and tries to make sense of—my father's
endless pacing, his desperate wandering, from room to room of our house.*

Wheeling My Father through the Alzheimer's Ward

EDWARD HIRSCH

Here where everyone forgets everything,
including where they are
or what they are fighting to remember,

I can't help recalling the childhood afternoon
that I was bloodied in a baseball game
by a kid who wanted to murder me,

and how my father, who was streetwise
to the world, a former Golden Gloves champ
in the lightweight division in west Chicago,

laced me into a pair of shiny red gloves
and then chalked a ring in our backyard,
shouting encouragement from the corner . . .

My old man taught me to raise my hands
and keep moving, to feint and weave,
to dance on the balls of my feet

and use my shoulders when I punched,
to stutter-step and lean, to jab hard
with my left, and hook with my right.

My father taught me never to be afraid
to fight, while I grunted and pranced
around our patio under the sweating lights,

bounding off the imaginary ropes
to defend myself, tasting my own blood,
shadowboxing an invisible enemy.

This poem is a parable of memory and forgetfulness. It links a story, an involuntary memory from childhood, with the experience of wheeling my father through the poignant Alzheimer's ward of a nursing home.

Home Care

DAVID MASON

My father says his feet will soon be trees
and he is right, though not in any way
I want to know. A regal woman sees
me in the hallway and has much to say,
as if we were lovers once and I've come back
to offer her a rose. But I am here
to find the old man's shoes, his little sack
of laundered shirts, stretch pants and underwear.

Rattling a metal walker for emphasis,
his pal called Joe has one coherent line—
How the hell they get this power over us?—
then logic shatters and a silent whine
crosses his face. My father's spotted hands
flutter like dying moths. I take them up
and lead him in a paranoiac dance
toward the parking lot and our escape.

He is my boy, regressed at eighty-two
to mooncalf prominence, drugged and adrift.
And I can only play, remembering who
he was not long ago, a son bereft.
Strapped in the car, he sleeps away the hour
we're caught in currents of the interstate.
He will be ashes in a summer shower
and sink to roots beneath the winter's weight.

*My father was the most adventurous man I have ever known, both physically
and emotionally, and to see him decline so precipitously in his final years was
often horrible. His wife, Claire Tangvald, bravely cared for him all that time, only*

occasionally putting him in a home to get some relief. This poem is a true story about one of those rare occasions when I was able to help out with this aspect of his care. At one point he really did look down at his feet and mumble, "They're gonna be trees."

We All Fall Down

NANCY DAHLBERG

Mother has fallen four times these past two weeks
as if she's drawn to the final position.
Stretched out on the floor, she's as close to the ground

as she can get in this home for the aged,
but no one will grant her wish for a return
to the earth—each time she falls the nurses call

an ambulance. The friendly paramedics say, "Irene,
you can't go on like this," and I think she hopes
it's true. Emergency room x-rays reveal

no fractures, but when she returns, I can see
that she's broken. Two weeks before she leaves us,
I manicure her fingernails, kneel to bathe

her blue-veined feet, hack at tough nails that belie
fragility; then towel and powder her toes
while she sits, and dozing answers, "Yes, that does

feel nice." On the floor I stroke her swollen feet
and weep over years thickened with memory.
This image remains: myself at fifty-five

trying to show my mother how love is felt
through the flesh; as if by caressing her feet
I could demonstrate the way to love a child.

*My mother was diagnosed with dementia in her mid-80s, when she began to
misinterpret and, later, detach herself from the details of this world. "We All Fall
Down" relays events in the last weeks of my mother's life as well as my attempt to
come to terms with the complexity of our changed relationship.*

Visiting Rose Haven Adult Family Home

DENISE CALVETTI MICHAELS

for Hugo Joseph Bianco, 1914–2005

The words he remembers are like remainders
of a long division problem we converted
to fractions in grade school, only a piece
of the whole, fragments, Mr. Fernandez,
our 4th grade teacher, proved to us, mean
　　—something remains, like scent of alfalfa.

Yesterday, my father's words float
on the water of memory
like lotus blossoms at moonrise
and I hear *his* father's
staccato voice
echo in the mirror
　　—*testa dura testa dura*
and the hard stones
of my father's childhood
rise from silt:
Paso Robles,
the ranch and family dairy,
the grove of oak that wept acorns to the ground.

I stand beside his bed and he sees Flora,
his cousin with long, dark hair,
not understanding three quarters of a century
have gone by since he teased her,
ran barefoot on the earth in Gonzalez,

my father, fine-boned, like a wren,
the remainder of a long division
into perfect circles,
concentric and widening,

carried on the skin of water,
the past, a dry river of stones
we throw back to break the water.

My poem begins in journal notes on the flight back home to Seattle after the first visit to see my father since his transition to Rose Haven. My visit, my presence, triggered his memory of the ranch where I was willing to go that day in May with him—acorns and alfalfa, alive, palpable like a dream I remember. "Testa dura" means hard head.

Equations

JAYNE PUPEK

I remember equations but not the name of my wife.
Years spent moving between desk and blackboard,

yellow chalk numbers in columns, the smell of textbooks
and pencil lead. Theorems raced across the page

like brilliant stars or musical notes. In those days,
I was a god, the grand conductor. I still feel the metal

protractor exacting a circle. Mathematics
explained all I needed to know: how much to add,

how much to take away. How to multiply and divide.
What to do with what remains.

Today, a nurse escorts visitors to my bed.
She assigns each one a name. This is your family,

she insists. Not students. The students are gone.
They stand around, a row of faces

waiting to see who I know. In the evening's dim light,
they are decimal points perfectly aligned.

In this poem, the subject loses details of his family members but recalls details from his work as a mathematics professor. At the end of the poem, the family members themselves converge into decimal points. I wanted to show how memory is lost in a piecemeal way, and the order is somehow random and unpredictable.

The Visit

KAY MULLEN

Take the side gate, the nurse says,
then the outer entrance
and down the hall to double doors
with the numbered key and flashing
green light to let you in. We find
my sister alone, sitting on the bed's edge,

her clasped hands shaking as if cupping
dice in a game of Yahtzee. She stares
with puzzled eyes, her mouth
waiting for words she strains to speak.
I hold her hand as we walk around the rose
courtyard more times than I can remember.

Back in her room I feed her ice cream
from a cone. We listen to Christmas carols
and Mozart. I dance as she sways
to the music, smiles. She told me once
she rescued me when we were children.
Now she can't remember why,

nor who it was she saved.

*My sister spent the last three years of her life in an Alzheimer's nursing home unit.
The gradual decline in her memory began in her early 60s. She died at 72. The
poem was written after one of my last visits with her.*

The Poem in Which the Histologist Learns the Meaning of Irony

MADELYN GARNER

You spent years
with a handheld steel blade
parting your Red Sea:
the hollow hearts of blastocysts.

How thinly
could you slice the living
world into Escher-like variations
for the electron microscope?

Unaware that in a parallel universe
your brain was shrinking:
billions of cells corrupted—
synapses amputated,
nuclei swept of meaning.

Now you are embedded
between the rails of a bed,
reduced to diagonal,
limbs stiffening
in Alzheimer's paraffin,
speech fragmented into fractals,

beyond knowing
how well you mastered
the narrows.

As a histologist, my sister was known for her superior technical skills and innovations. It took doctors two years to diagnose her Alzheimer's; during that time she spent nights alone in the lab checking and reprocessing each day's output to assure the accuracy of her research work. Amazing.

Recognition

KATE BERNADETTE BENEDICT

How tranquil it is, sitting here with my witless mother
who does not recognize me.
I brush and braid her long white silken hair.

When I take her hand, she laces her fingers in my fingers.
Then she sings: *cockles and mussels, alive alive oh.*

She does not remember her marriage of forty years.
She does not mourn the husband she cannot name.
The drunken struggles, the blaming, the carping—
nothing of severity remains.

When a car door slams outside,
she tells me her papa has come to deliver her.
I'll take you home again, Kathleen.

"Kitty has company," a nurse announces, entering the room.
"Company," my mother echoes. "O, please stay for tea."

To me the nurse whispers:
"She acts like a queen, so that's how we treat her."
She, who waved an imperial arm to no avid throng, a queen?

When her eyes close and her head bows,
we take a nap together in her slender bed.

How restful it is, lying here this August day
with my witless mother,
this mother I prize and do not recognize.

"Catherine," the jaunty Maine caregivers would say to my mother when I visited, "don't you recognize your daughter?" While I appreciated their good intentions, inwardly I'd flinch. I had come to respect my mother's addlement and didn't want her confused further by insistent questions about my identity. "Identity" had become a slippery concept in the wake of my mother's illness and "recognition" an issue for us both.

Confirmation

NANCY DAHLBERG

Her own door locked, key neon-spiraled on her wrist,
Mother roams the rooms of the nursing home,
accuses fellow residents of stealing her incontinence pads,
Madeira cookies, scatter pins, anything she can't remember
having used or eaten or squirreled away. Yesterday,
to gray heads bobbing over Cream of Wheat and runny eggs,
she complained that her children wrote large checks on her account,
have stolen her money, then hinted no one there is safe,
poison could be in the food. Mary choked
and dropped her orange juice, arthritic Leota
refused to swallow the Nuprin, and the manager called
with, please, we need another talk. *Lies,*
my mother says, *all lies,* then weeps and mutters
her curse: *The rest of you should live to be so old.*
Every day she gives the office two weeks' notice
she's moving back to the old neighborhood
where she can walk to what she needs, even though
a walk to the door exhausts her and once outside,
she's lost. Mother can't remember she forgot to eat
and ended up at Lutheran General, a mirrored counter
where her sofa should have been, the trees outside
replaced by a five-story building; and after
she went home, her own room's strange.
Nothing remembered, not even the old photographs
I unboxed, thinking at least she had her past.
That day I handed her the portrait of herself at twelve,
head tilted toward white-flounced shoulder,
one hand on her hip, full lips closed in a smile.
Is this Maggie? she frowned, referring to my youngest daughter,
and turning the picture over, read the strong slanted hand
on the back—"Irene, 1914, Confirmation." *My mother*

wrote that, she said, and pleased this time, looked
again at the young girl, her pale eyes bright.

"Confirmation" tells of the events and mental confusion that led to my mother's being ousted from an assisted living facility and her subsequent transfer to a full-care nursing home.

Within His Grasp

MARION BOYER

When he's nervous my father whistles,
tuneless as a radiator. The window
sections his world down to a patch
like a framed photograph. The crossbeams

in his head refuse to hold whatever version
of me he knew. At times his hands work
a delicate apparatus only visible to him
as though he labors over a small knot,

repairing dragonfly wings. Other moments
his hands lift to capture whatever floats
in the remainder of his mind, perhaps
the slow waltz of blown seed pods

from twelve summers ago. He smoothes
his trousers, brushes imaginary lint
or tugs at a tiny piece of skin on his lip.
They are the slender fingers

of an accountant who shifted numbers
from column to column as someone
more ancient than he slid beads on an abacus.
Now he worries a bit of blanket fluff

into a small bramble. I reach over
with a fork of cold potato for his mouth
and his hand clamps the wheelchair arm
with such strength I remember he is still a man.

My father has suffered with Alzheimer's for the past 10 years. We've lost my father's mother and my husband's mother to this disease as well. I wrote this poem after one of my visits to see him in the nursing home where he's been a resident for the past five years.

Hands

MARGOT WIZANSKY

He is surprised by his hands,
observes them seriously, brings
one hand up to his face, long cold
purple fingers, knurled arthritic joints.
He places one against the other,
pressing finger to finger in an arch.
His hands remember all the ways
they've ever moved, swiveling at the wrists
as though they're leading an orchestra,
appearing to thread a needle and soar,
gliding sideways across the luncheon tray
as once I watched him check the buff
and polish of a Queen Anne chest.
All the while we play Bach for him
and stare—old, old man, his hands
that come to rest, one hand curled
around my mother's finger as an infant
grasps in reflex, love's first and last.

"Hands" was written after a wonderful visit with my stepfather, whose Alzheimer's was quite advanced. He was unable to speak but listened to his favorite classical music and conducted. With his hands, he acted out work he had done in the past, furniture building, upholstering. He still had kinetic memory.

Sarcophagus

HOLLY ZEEB

Side by side
hands entwined
my mother and I
recline on
her narrow bed
keep company
with the spirits
emanating
from photographs
of ancestors
Japanese prints
beloved objects
from her past
lives
Eyes closed
we breathe in unison
suspended
for a time
I forget
her forgetting
Her fingers
in mine
slender
long
familiar

For many years I have written poems about my mother's progressive dementia—to record what she seems to be experiencing, to grieve her losses and my own, and to sustain myself as I become her memory. As her language and memory have disappeared, we have become oddly more intimate physically.

VIII.
Missing Pieces

Night

SHEBANA COELHO

Every night before going to bed, she presents herself to him, head bowed. If not for the two women holding her elbows, she would not be upright. As it is, she hunches, an inverted comma.

In his white kurta, he stands, ready for her. It is the most focused thing he does each day. Other times, he is lost in the murky grey of his eyes.

So she presents herself to him. They meet in the middle of the room, in a no-man's-land with the sitting area behind her and the dining area behind him. Usually the TV is playing very loudly and the two servants sometimes glance back at it because the show that they were watching is not yet over.

So she presents herself to him, head bowed. He cups her face with his hands and kisses the top of her head. He has long knobby fingers. They almost meet at the back of her head. She turns her head into his hand. Usually she turns to the right but sometimes to the left. So she turns into either hand and then takes it into her own. She kisses his knuckles. There are dusts of powder on the nape of her neck. He kisses the back of her hand, the hand that encloses his. She wavers. The servants tighten their hold. He kisses her hand again. All the while, they are saying goodnight to each other. Her litany is at times soft and at times harsh because she cannot control her modulation. His litany is loud and certain, a promise of better times ahead. He says *Allah madat karo*, may god help us, and that is usually the signal for them to part.

The servants lead her into her room, an artificial room that used to be a storeroom but now has been completely made up into a sickroom with a hospital bed that can raise or lower her. The bed has a metal railing so she doesn't get up in the middle of the night and run away from the illness that has consumed her so quickly.

He goes to his room, once their room that used to long ago have a large double bed and now has two single beds because he snored too loudly, and she had to go to the bathroom too often, and so it was thought that two separate beds on either side of the room would allow them to fully indulge these behaviors without aggravating the other.

Past the foot of the beds, against the wall is a three-column dresser: a vertical strip of mirror edged by two columns of drawers. At the base of the mirror, a shelf that holds artifacts of younger days: lipsticks and eyeliners and jewelry—all manner of necklaces with beads from the factory they owned. On the floor in front of this mirror is a faint ring, an outline of a short, wicker stool that used to be there for many years. The stool is now in the front room—she uses it to rest her feet as she seesaws from upright to supine on the daybed where she spends, what else, her days.

I have memories of her sitting on that stool, in front of that dresser, carefully applying a dark rose lipstick and some blush. Her smile, when she caught me watching, would come sudden and quick, and I would falter for a second before smiling back.

She would sometimes lower her voice and say: *you know, I forget easily so keep reminding me okay.* She'd speak in a whisper and what I registered was that she was taking me into her confidence, not that she was forgetting. What I registered was her telling me where she hid this bit of money or where she stored that bit of jewelry.

Now as she is forgetting more and more, I am remembering more and more. I am remembering the tiny blips, the small flickers along the way. I am remembering that she held a torch ahead of us and pointed to things on the walls, drawings and paintings of the birds and the animals and the people that now she alone can see.

This piece describes a nightly ritual between my grandmother, who has Alzheimer's, and my grandfather, who does not. About four months after her sudden and rapid descent into the disease, I visited them in India. She was in that space where what she had been could still be discerned amid what she was becoming. I didn't plan on writing anything but on my return, woke up one morning with vivid images of their "goodnights" and so recorded them.

Missing Pieces
January 18, 1998

DIANE PORTER GOFF

4:20 A.M.—Mama raps again on our bedroom door—the fifth time tonight. The raps are loud and sharp, so I know her anxiety is up, despite the pills I have given her earlier. My husband groans and rolls over. I drag myself to the door, and Mama is standing in the weak light of the hall, a diminutive figure with a suitcase. She has put on two pairs of pajama tops with her bra fastened over them. She wears brown wool pants with her black snow boots on the wrong feet, so that her toes stick out at ridiculous angles. On her head is her broad-brimmed traveling hat. If it weren't so sad, I'd have to laugh.

"I want to go home," she announces in a troubled voice. Her eyes dart fearfully around the hall.

"Mama, you are home. You live here now with me and Richard and Larkin." I stroke her arm. "See your room and your cozy bed?"

She jerks her arm away. "Stop trying to fool me. I've got to get home. My mama is waiting for me. She doesn't know where I am. She'll be worried. She's waiting for me." Her brow furrows and her lower lip trembles.

"Mama, you can't go home just now. You . . ."

She turns toward the stairs. "I AM going now. I want to go HOME."

I catch her before she starts down. "OK, you can go, but let's get your clothes on right. You don't want to go home without your sweater and coat. Your clothes are a little mixed up. And don't you want to go to the bathroom before you go?" I'm hoping to break this traveling trend.

She stares at me suspiciously, and then relents. "OK, I'll go to the bathroom."

I leave her alone for a minute, then return. "It's alright." I announce in a bright voice, "I've called your mother and she wants you to wait until daylight to come home. Let's just lie down till then."

"She isn't worried?"

"No, I told her you are coming at daylight. Let's lie down."

She leans heavily on my arm on the way back to bed. I help her get her pajamas on right.

"Do you want me to lie down with you for a while?" I ask.

"Yes, please." Her voice is like a tired child's.

We lie there, side by side. All my cells seem to sag with weariness, but I can't sleep. I watch her profile, the high forehead, the strongly arched nose. I think of the many times I have studied its strength, know how much it comforts me, even now at this strange time in our lives.

Suddenly she turns to me. "Do you have a mother?" She whispers confidentially.

"Yes, I have a mother." I finally whisper back.

"Where is she?"

For a moment I cannot speak. Grief lies like a small stone against my lips.

Then I take a breath and answer. "My mother is waiting for me, too." I reply. "Somewhere, she's waiting for me."

My sister Beverly and I cared for Mama through five years of Alzheimer's, dividing her time between my home in Virginia and my sister's home in Georgia. Our first clue that something was amiss was Mama not being able to keep up with her checkbook and with my father's sudden death, she spiraled rapidly downward into the disease. The journey was long and arduous—sometimes so funny it broke us up, sometimes so sad, it seemed to literally break our hearts.

Saturdays with Mom

BARBARA S. SIMPSON

The fight started small. I was curling my hair. She took my brush, said it was hers. I took it back. She called me a thief and a shit, said she hated and wanted to kill me. I said, "Yeah, Mom, I know." I'd heard it before.

She grabbed the brush again. I grabbed it back and slapped it down on the sink. She snatched it and bared her unbrushed teeth in a demented grin. I pried her fingers loose—she was incredibly strong—and jerked the brush out of her hand. "Dammit, Mom, can't you leave me alone for five minutes?" Her dark eyes snapped up and down the way they always had when she was angry. Somehow, I no longer found it funny. "Fine! If you want it, take it!" I said and threw the brush against the wall.

It didn't hit her, didn't even come close, but it startled her into action. Gone was the woman who loved birds and babies and cantaloupe with chocolate ice cream, gone the woman my aunts called "drill sergeant." In her place was a screeching bird-woman who swooped at me, mouth open, fingers curled. I threw up my arms. She grabbed me. Held on. Shrieked. One jagged fingernail ripped into my hand. I screamed and shoved her. She fell, hard. Her collection of glass bells jangled.

I stood there, breathing hard, crying from pain and shame and expended rage, blood dripping from my hand. She cowered on one hip, mewling like a wounded animal, one arm raised to protect herself. She was no longer some fierce creature with hot eyes but a frightened, confused old woman in an aqua sweat suit, unable to get up on her own. I wiped my face on my flannel shirt. Tears fell as I braced my feet, bent over, and began the nearly impossible task of hauling her upright.

I wish I could say that was the only—or even the last—time I lost my temper. And that I did enough to help my father during the years he cared for Mom. What I can tell you is this: with elderly or ailing parents, there is no "enough."

And that you have to look within for absolution.

It was a Saturday sometime in the '80s. I don't remember when, exactly; my mother's deterioration from Alzheimer's disease lasted many years, and it's hard to remember what happened when. I only know it was a Saturday because that was my day to stay with her.

Reprieve

TINA WELLING

Tonight, after my mother's steady breathing assures me she is fast asleep, I sneak out to the living room. I open a window and breathe in humid, fragrant air, grateful that Mom is asleep and won't complain about the breezes. I listen to crickets and night birds. Then turn on a reading lamp and get comfortable with my book and my solitude.

Ten minutes pass. Is that a doorknob turning? I decide that it isn't and return to my book. Suddenly, my mother appears in the living room. She is fully dressed. She has not dressed herself for a year.

"Good morning," she says. She looks quite refreshed for having only fifteen minutes' sleep. And she looks beautiful. Intelligent and cheerful. She looks familiar. The dread I felt at having my time interrupted glides smoothly into pure delight at seeing her remembered face.

"Aw," I say, hating to disappoint her, "it's not morning. It's still nighttime."

"Hmm?"

"Oh, never mind. Come sit with me." I pat the cushion next to me.

She walks around the coffee table and sits on the sofa beside me. She looks at my face a long moment, then says, "You know, you are very pretty. There's just something about you . . . something special."

I say, "Thank you. You always make me *feel* special. That's why you are such a wonderful mother to me." At the word mother, I almost lose her. Her eyes slip focus a second before she regains her composure. I warn myself not to ruin this time for us, to be careful of what I say. But I don't want to heed my warning; I am with my lifetime best friend and we are telling each other important things.

She notices my flowered nightgown and admires it.

"Daddy gave this to me for my birthday."

"Oh? Do you know Daddy?"

"Yes . . . I do." I stop myself from saying more.

"Well, imagine that!" She marvels over my knowing my own father, but I smooth that away in my mind. My whole being soaks up her presence. So many nights since I was a young girl she and I have sat like this—the sounds of Bessie Creek lapping at the dock, the occasional croak of the pig frog, the mottled duck's squawk drifting in to us and mingling with our confidences. This is the gift of one more night. I don't want it to end.

My mother looks relaxed and happy. She notices the opened window. "Goodness, it's black out there. What's that say?" She points to the clock.

"Eight-thirty."

"What in the world are we doing up?" With the expression familiar to me as a prelude to joking, my mother raises her eyebrows, gives me her impish look, and says, "One of us is crazy."

Art and healing are natural partners. The essay "Reprieve" began as a journal entry in an attempt to heal myself from the confusion and contradictions presented during my mother's struggle with Alzheimer's disease. The process of crafting the entry into an essay broadened the personal into the universal. The final transformation of the writing resulted in a fictional scene in my novel, Crybaby Ranch, *which turned the story into the lives of any mother and any daughter facing change, illness, endings. Healing often creates art; art often creates healing.*

Eclipse

MARY BARRETT

The more incompetent Dad became, the more I liked him. His loss of memory, especially his loss of precise, exacting language, changed everything about how we related. He'd had a brilliant legal mind and corrected me constantly. He impatiently demanded to know what I meant by what I had, in his mind, so sloppily said. He'd challenge, and I'd feel angry and hurt. He never just listened for my meaning; it seemed my choice of words could evict me from his good graces.

Now I could relax around him because it didn't matter anymore how I said things. The gate to his loving heart, so rigidly defended by legal correctness, had burst open. There were no more ego boundaries, no fences, no rock walls; Alzheimer's had made him as soft and accessible as ripe fruit.

One summer before he died, my children and I spent a hot August month with him in sticky upstate New York. There was to be an eclipse and a blood red moon, so I carted a rickety lawn chair outside for him. The children and I sat on blankets around him under a huge maple. We watched for endless dragging minutes as the earth passed though the sun's path and crept over the moon's brightness.

Dad sat in his green sports jacket, his Irish peaked cap, his slacks and tie shoes and watched us, oblivious to the point. He asked repeatedly why we were out there, what were we doing? Then he'd laugh when we said we were watching the moon.

"Oh, I forgot," he said.

He sat with us for the entire eclipse, while my son turned somersaults on the grass, and my daughter yawned and strained to stay awake. As the moon regained its light, we sang every moon song he'd taught me—"Shine on Harvest Moon," "Moonlight Bay," "The Moon Belongs to Everyone." He bellowed out lyrics he hadn't yet forgotten. I never felt so close to him.

After my mother died, it became clear my father was unable to remember anything on his own. I spent many weeks with him and had a mix of emotions so strong that usual outlets couldn't handle them, so I wrote my first poems trying to work through those feelings. "Eclipse" was written as a little piece remembered years later during the anniversary of his death.

Naked

SYBIL LOCKHART

The day of her physical, my mother is wearing the same dirty, rumpled clothes she's worn the past four times I've seen her. Ma wears her greasy blue hat with the earflaps down. Her glasses, speckled with spots of food and flaked skin, cause her to peer out squintingly, scrunching up her nose as she rushes headlong into the hospital room. She hurries to undress even after I remind her that this doctor always keeps her waiting a minimum of twenty minutes. She grunts, knees popping, as she bends to remove each shoe, and each loose, grey sock. "Dzok!" my daughter Cleo reports from her stroller; "Sheoo!!" Ma's fraying cargo pants fall to the floor in a crumpled pile, and she steps out, then gently folds them.

I glance uneasily about, my eyes avoiding her body. I have anticipated and avoided this moment. I've been watching the steady degradation of Ma's personality: The Loss Of. The loss of passion, the loss of opinions, of esteem, of self-esteem; the loss of self. I'm afraid of seeing my old mom so vulnerable, so weak: naked. I fear the sight of her sagging, flaccid, spotted flesh. At the same time, I regard her body with a morbid fascination. It shocks, it unearths me, to experience this slow but monumental shift from my laughing, competent, mother to a passive, humorless stranger. Her body will give me confirmation of her mind's deterioration, I think, when I witness that fragile old skeleton drooping with the flesh of the infirm.

So I look. And I look again, surprised. Her legs are full and alive. Their fleshy, muscled thighs and calves are shaped familiarly like my own. Something shifts inside me.

As she removes her bra, her fingers calmly following a course set by many decades of habit, she seems to give her nakedness before me about as much thought as Cleo does when I change her diaper. Out of Ma's bra emerge two full, round breasts, several sizes larger than mine, just as they always have been: big, earthy breasts. Why did I expect wrinkled tubular sacks hanging down to her bellybutton?

There she stands, a still-attractive, shapely woman. She stoops only slightly. Without her clothes, she is fully physical, generously feminine. Her grey hair falls sweetly to her shoulders as she slips into the blue gown. She climbs onto the doctor's table, tissue paper crackling under her, and leans back with a sigh, and I surge with renewed affection. My mother has grace; she has a natural, innocent composure. Her animal body has an ease that her worried mind no longer possesses. Her yellow chipped teeth, her greying hair, her muddied thoughts, cannot override the simple, beautiful fact of her womanhood.

I was at home with my two young children when my mother was diagnosed with Alzheimer's disease. My girls helped to refill the well, not just by cheering up the gloomy moments but also by loving their grandma without judgment. I am also a member of a wonderful group of Berkeley writers called Motherlode. Writing and talking with them about child rearing, caregiving, and everything in between saved me again and again.

The Day Room

CHRISTINE HIGGINS

I go to see my mother in the nursing home. It's Christmastime, so naturally they have an Italian tenor singing *Ave Maria* and a little girl from my old grade school singing *Silent Night*. I wheel my mother up close to my folding chair, and I say, *You have such a beautiful voice.* She no longer remembers my name or who I am, but she can sing all the words to *O Come All Ye Faithful*. She lifts her twisted hand and shields her eyes the way she used to after she took communion. A little while later, she turns to me and says, *Bill is coming to take me shopping.* Then, in twirl the middle-aged ladies in tap shoes and red-and-white-checked aprons, clicking their feet to the beat of a Hungarian folk song. When they twirl, the fat jiggles beneath their pink satin cheeks. The room is festooned with gold and silver garland, and all the employees are smiling.

I want to find the Chinese woman who isn't allowed in the day room. I know she's up on the second floor, strapped into a high-backed chair that converts into a bed. She is banging the metal table with her fist and screaming.

My father kept my mother at home with him for as long as he could. Two years after her diagnosis, he could no longer manage, and we found a nursing home close to where they lived. "The Day Room" takes place during the first Christmas she was there, when we went to visit her and found everyone gathered for the entertainment.

In Which Grandma Belle Navigates the Altoona Nursing Home

NINA CORWIN

Grandma Belle wanders the sanitized hallways, looking for the next flight out. Somehow, she manages to slip off the unit and negotiates her way unnoticed to the lobby on the main floor. Once there, she sees a red-haired receptionist with an operator's headset guarding the glass doors that tease her with freedom just a few steps away.

Looks like one of those *schikse* airline reservation types, she thinks as she struggles to remember a destination that might make her welcome. Maybe London. Or Amsterdam. The people were nice there. But the point is she's looking for a flight to reunite her with her sister, her mother, her husband, all the ones who've left ahead. Except somehow, her son, who she forgets, thirteen years gone; something no mother should have to live through, much less remember. Forgetting is so much easier now.

Approaching the counter, she asks the price of a one-way ticket, and the receptionist plays along, not wanting to be the one to undress a dream. Instead she quotes a ticket price impossibly high, and Belle, ever the *balboosteh*, wheedles the woman, the art of the bargain still embedded in her very chromosomes.

"Oy, such prices! The agents upstairs aren't nearly so expensive," she lies without blinking an eye. It's the oldest gambit in the book. But the headset woman's heard that one before. Saw the likes of it in a book of Yiddish wit and wisdom she read for a class in multiculturalism at the community college up the way. "So, why don't you buy it from them?" she counters, pleased as a punch line right on time.

Belle doesn't have ready access to a good response, or to her social security checks, on direct deposit to a bank impossibly far away, maybe Manhattan. Beyond reach. For a moment, the wiry hairs twitch quietly above her upper lip.

Then, tottering on eighty-nine years of tired limbs, she picks her withered way toward the gleaming Mop & Glo institutional steel elevators. Up, down, whatever. She only wants they should carry her anywhere but the urine-scented barracks on which they've assigned her a bed. A candy striper finds her; and worries, with a condescending hand upon her gaunt shoulder, that "Grandma" might get lost. To which Belle quips, "This is an elevator. How lost can I get?"

And yet beyond, it could all be anywhere. Some sort of Limbo just one level up from that Dante-esque final destination. And she knows with the only certainty given her; she's got to get a seat on the next flight out.

Like so many others, my grandmother never wanted to find herself in a nursing home. She was a strong, even intimidating little woman; a Russian immigrant become teacher in the New York City Schools throughout her working life. Although I have taken some liberties in this telling, I have attempted to render her spirit and experience, a tough survivor struggling for mastery over that stage at which one has least control of one's own life.

Kaddish

SARAH LEAVITT

When my mother, Midge, got Alzheimer's at the age of 53, the rabbi taught me the prayer that Moses said to God when God struck Miriam with leprosy: *El na refah na la*—Heal her Lord, please heal her. I said the prayer every day, even though there was no possibility of healing. I never found a prayer for the terminally ill, and during her long death I envied the mourners who recited the kaddish—a prayer that was meant exactly for them and that marked a definite ending.

At first my mother fought hard against the disease, with a resilience that was as much a part of her as her tall, strong body, her potent sparking anger and bitter sense of humor. Then she stopped being able to remember or understand dates, or comprehend the passage of time, so my age and birthday were a mystery to her. She lost the concept of mother and daughter. She stopped saying my name. She asked me who I was. She did not respond at all when I entered the room. These were all deaths, weren't they? Or one long, slow death. Imagine if there were a prayer for every stage in a long death.

She grew less and less able to care for herself. We helped her bathe and dress. And then we started coming into the bathroom with her, pulling down her pants, helping her onto the toilet, wiping her. We stripped the sheets and bathed her after she wet the bed, wiped her nose, cleaned food from her chin. She wandered the house blank-faced, humming.

After seven years she died.

I said the kaddish, that prayer I had wanted, but it didn't fit. The prayer praises God, who my mother never believed in anyway.

Allen Ginsberg's poem "Kaddish" was written in honor of his mother, Naomi, after he learned that no one had said kaddish at her funeral. Naomi died in a psychiatric hospital after years of suffering from mental illness. Ginsberg remembers his mother not as the woman she was before her breakdowns but as she was in illness:

Blessed be you Naomi in tears!
Blessed be you Naomi in fears!
    Blessed Blessed Blessed in sickness!
. . .

Blest be your last years' loneliness!
Blest be your failure! Blest be your stroke! Blest be the
close of your eye! Blest be the gaunt of your cheek!
Blest be your withered thighs!

When I think of my mother, now burnt into ashes, I remember the hairs under her chin and the thin scar at the base of her spine and the ripples of varicose veins on her thighs and her dry peeling feet. The thick blue veins on her hands, her large ears, her bitten nails. The things that I was never supposed to know so intimately. I miss the mother I tucked into bed, the mother I bathed and dressed and fed as if she were my child. "Blessed be you Midge in confusion!" I say to her. "Blessed be you Midge in shame! Blest be your last years' nakedness! Blest be your forgetting! Blest be your memory!"

My mother, Midge Leavitt, died in November 2004 at the age of 60. She was a bright, healthy woman, and the disease hit her out of the blue; she had no family history and none of the suspected risk factors. I spent as much time as I could with her while she was ill, though we lived on opposite sides of the country. Her illness is what motivated me to become serious about my writing; I recorded as much as I could about her illness, and since her death writing has helped me to hang onto her in some small way.

IX.
Here Let Us

Here Let Us
Late Middle Alzheimer's Disease

DONNA WAHLERT

Here let us sit together
under the weeping beech
here let us talk about milk glass
chifforobes and elderberry wine
here let us soothe your ankles
swollen with childhood memories
we won't remind you that your mother
has been gone for thirty years
that the house you want to go
home to is no longer there
that your children are grown and gray
that you are the last of your friends
here let us drink our wintergreen tea
and talk about this primrose
the thin spaghetti you had for lunch
the nurse who brings you Hershey bars
here let us not dream about the days to come
here let us sing you your mother
here let us sing you your children
here let us sing you home.

In the eighth year of her Alzheimer's disease, I wheeled my mother outside under a shady tree. As we shared the moment, I realized that for Mother there was no longer any past, and she was unable to contemplate the future. I realized then that all we had was this present moment.

Prayer for My Mother

RICK KEMPA

Let every moment of every day
break upon her with the dazzle of
utter newness, and let her exult in it.

Let wonder rule: the sky more lovely
than she's ever seen, the birds that
come by the hundred to her feeder.

Please let her forget that she does not
remember. Let her lose somehow
the torment of losing her mind.

Let there be insight in the one page that,
over and over for days, she reads
for the first time, never gets beyond.

Let the living past be vibrant in her
dreams each night, her mother, her brother
at her side, showering her with love.

Please let her eyes open in the morning
not to the despair of the lost at sea,
but to the familiar play of sunlight

in the leaves outside her window,
the solid sense that she is safe,
the firm ground of home.

*For nearly two years, until she moved to a nursing home, my mother lived with
my wife, our two teenage children, and me. Her presence was a gift: we coalesced
around her, sharing the pleasure of her boundless love, the challenges of being her
caregivers, and the sadness as her health declined.*

Returning Thanks

JOEL A. MCCOLLOUGH

For seventy years his prayers ran long,
sonorous in the waspy rafters
of his Baptist preacher's palate.
We bent dirty necks and fidgeted,
three grandsons dunce-stooled
down the kitchen counter
in order of descending birthdays,
slavering at piled platters
of fried chicken and tater tots
in plastic wicker baskets.

We clasped and prayed for amen.

Which comes too quickly now
and seems to ask forgiveness
for what went before.
At dinner you squeezed my hand
as I counted just six words,
cadent as the King James
but unmoored from syntax,
alone and floating like the peaks
of a country almost submerged.

A spare blessing that does not keep us.

In "Returning Thanks," I record the peculiarly Southern sacrament of a family dinner, hosted by my grandparents, of fast-food fried chicken. My grandfather was a gifted public speaker and asked the blessing at all family gatherings. The diminution of his verbal faculties was the first sign most of us had of the onset of the disease.

Elegy / in advance / do not hasten

DAN BELLM

1.

Caught—between the prayer for healing and the prayer
For the dead—most unappeasable and un-
Consoled remembrances—the words I need
The most, and cannot say—*hineini*—I am here,
The nowhere man, and I address no one
Unceasingly—What meanings will be carried
Over for us now, and who will hear—
Tell me—No One—now that, mother to son,
No more remembrance is to be allowed—
And who will recognize us as we are?—
I am undone by minutes—I am undone
By days—mother—taking her hand—afraid
What to ask—doubtful what to pray—
Remembering—as she pulls her hand away—

2.

Mystery visitor of the constantly strange moment,
mother
of disappearingness,
sitting in church without her memory—

what to do with these fretful hands
but fold them together O God—

Quieting herself
among the knots and tangles,
dropped threads, the clutter
of self and unself she once
would have cleared away,

and answering what half-heard voices of before
cross her face with strickenness—

household saint
who swept the room and prepared the food and served it,
then stood to one side so the men
could do their work,

humble Martha, handmaiden of the Lord
with her reticent smile, her
pale private frown—

*

Sometimes we sit
and lose our memory together,
I can almost stop presuming I
am here,
each turning of time becoming
the purest other,
the questions not asked remaining where they are—

Sometimes we worry the surfaces of things,
she tears at scars and bruises on her face,
has to be taken by the hand—

Holding hands I think
I am becoming her,
as we must have been not separate once
if there was heaven,
one single fate of lostness to come, if there is not,

and what tears do I mean to drag out of her this way
with the smallest tenderness,
for my own wishing—
will I snap her out of it, since I am also Dad,
shake her and say, *Let's scream our little heads off,*
fly off the fucking handle together for once—

for what—
she doesn't know who I am—

*

Sometimes she mentions her *first husband*
and there was only one,
sounding like someone she maybe liked a little better—

*

She hums—
sits at the window for someone to arrive
and take her
home—*one of my children—*
leaving any day now,
someone else can have that room—
she hums,

as you might do if you don't have a word
or stop knowing how,
not even so you would hear
unless everything paused,
a solitary
conversation you might have no part in, a refrain,
nodding so very often to agree or remember to be there and the air
that breathes
you don't have to think about,
if you had a thought
you could let it cross your face
if somebody speaks,
or sings what you would
sing, a little shine,
or was to sit by your side
with a light in his eye
that if you loved me
you wouldn't want to hasten,

or hasten,
or bid me,
or adieu—

This poem partly arose from a conversation with my rabbi. At our synagogue, we say a prayer for the ill that asks for "a complete healing of body and spirit." Often, we agreed, this is not the right prayer. "Hineini" (Hebrew for "here I am") is the response made by Abraham, Isaac, Moses, and other Biblical figures to calls from God, a parent, or both.

X.

Time with the Dying

The suitcase propped open

ELIZABETH GARTON SCANLON

and on the bed, pitching heaps of crisp linen
on good hangers, cabled cotton, murky silks

testament to our reckless whimsy (*a few more
nighties,* my grandmother says, holding a tangle

of five, only one of which—wintry and long-sleeved—
I set aside.) *Three white nighties,* I write, *and one peach*

with lace in careful blue script as my mother's done
and my aunts each summer since they decided

it was folly leaving her to pack alone, dutifully
halving her piles, loading a sensible suitcase or two

into the back of the car, Grammy buckled in front
dozing, coral lipstick creamy and thick. This June

it is my turn, but I fill three bags, zippers straining,
and there is more, Grammy says, *jewelry . . . and scarves.*

Nine maybe ten weeks at the cottage—she doesn't
need all this, I know—but we cannot stop, giddy birds

pulling vivid threads and batting
for unnecessary nests. Still, I keep up the list

I've been told to (*three pairs of espadrilles, a watery
blouse*) as if afraid these bright things will get away

from us once we leave the house.

Every summer my grandparents traveled to their windswept family cottage on the shores of Lake Michigan. As Grammy began her drift into Alzheimer's, it became increasingly challenging but evermore important that she make the trip. One June I took a turn getting her ready to go. It was my last lucid time alone with her, and we giggled together over fabric and baubles and bags.

Moving Day, the Alzheimer's Wing

MARION BOYER

Today, we're a clothespin family. We admire
wallpaper, coax pleasantness onto the cloth
of our faces. We hang my father's watercolors,

pretend it's temporary. My mother and I paste
words in the air. He gazes through a window
across Chicago, the lake, and Michigan's cuff,

clear to Canada where he'll try to run. We move
clothes like we're setting out the Wedgwood,
or placing silverware precisely, nothing touching.

Here, the hallways are pressurized so smells
won't escape the rooms and residents'
doorways are marked with their faces framed

in construction paper. We're encouraged to think
of a shape that would represent my father.
Mr. Vanderoost is taped inside a blue windmill.

*It has been profoundly heartbreaking to see the many ways Alzheimer's diminishes
the personhood of my father. Although well-intentioned, it was painful to be asked
to further reduce him to a paper cutout representation.*

Moving My Mother

CATHLEEN CALBERT

She has her own place
in New York City

or southern California
by a red sun, a warm beach.

She hasn't lost her mind yet,
hasn't lost her apartment

in Berkeley, hasn't lost control
over her own body, isn't lying

alone in a nursing home in Chico,
a city that was never her own,

banging her ring against the rail
to see if anybody's listening.

I wish I could say that "Moving My Mother" is a persona poem, but the truth is it's a personal narrative prompted by the dreams I had once my mother ended up in a nursing home close to other family members. In this facility, the patients, including my mother, had one refrain: When will I go home? When do I get out of here? *Unable to help her flee what was a Kafkaesque descent into helplessness, I moved my mother, in my dreams, to another place and a time before Alzheimer's took control of her mind and body.*

After a Trip to the VA Hospital
Alzheimer's Ward, Tucson

JEFF WORLEY

Yesterday my mother tried for the third time
in seven months to finally "take Dad somewhere."
He'd agreed to this, she said. He'd agree, now,
to eat night crawlers if someone asked him.
I imagine my father there, unsteady on his cane,

thinking the doctor smiled like the dungeon man
in charge of leg irons, the nurse surely an actress
playing a nurse, everybody in on it,
Dad's new cellmate embellished with tubes,
eyes like marbles turned up from a ditch . . .

Back home, Mother tossed the suitcase on Dad's bed.
Put your things away yourself, she told him, snapping
open the luggage. *I'm tired of this.* Her anger
has traveled a long, slow fuse.

Later, talking to me on the portable, she recounts
his loud *Peg! Peg! Peggy!* as the doctor reached
to take him, how that broke her again.
Then she says she hears bathwater running.

She finds the carefully ironed shirts, terry cloth robe
and plaid house slippers floating in the tub,
Dad's voice from somewhere almost ghostlike:
Is this what you had in mind? Is this what you want?

*My father started showing signs of dementia around 1992, and he died from
Alzheimer's-related complications in October 2000. My father, a World War II*

veteran and former POW, spent a fair amount of time at the VA in Tucson, where they had a wing of rooms for people with dementia. But this was just a "transitional" solution: all patients had to be relocated to a larger care facility of some kind within two weeks. My mother tried to admit him at the VA, but my father—confused and scared—simply refused to be "turned over" the first time she tried.

The day after Auntie moves to The Maples

NANCY TUPPER LING

her Chester A. Reed Field Guide remains on the kitchen sill
overlooking the feeder. Inside, she recorded each sighting
in Palmer fashion. The common ones, finch and chickadee,
received a check mark like those given her best students
for jobs well done. But the rare birds ranked; their places
and dates inscribed like visiting guests. Twice in '76
she spotted the yellow-shafted flicker, his *wicker-wicker-
wicker* sounds. Under *Cedar Waxwing,* she noted the time
he stuffed himself madly with Papa's Tuftonboro berries.
Red juices dripping from beak. I, too, remember the day
we sat on Cuttyhunk's shore. Tourists slowly boarded
The Alert for the mainland while northern waterthrush
zipped about like Sandpipers between the piers, tracing
wavy outlines on the sand.

How did she know the short-eared owl, his pale buffy
breast in the snow? *Found, after a lifelong search.*
How did she know this silent stalker when her niece's name
had long been forgotten?

*When I discovered my great-aunt's field guide, all the memories of her watching
and recording the birds came back to me. Even when she couldn't put our names
with our faces, she still could name the beloved birds outside of her nursing home
window.*

Following the Deer

JOANNE CLARKSON

for Louise

Her vacant eyes reflect a square of blackberries

　Beyond the window
　Entwined in a hedge of weeds.
I bend to deliver the insulin, the quick sting
　As of bees searching for sweet vital juice.

She responds only with a whimper.
　I touch her shoulder and tell her
　She is brave.

Turning, I notice movement outside:
　Two does nibble blackberries,
Craning soft necks to avoid thorn, bees,
　Muzzles quivering.

"Look, Louise," I tell her, "there are deer."
　She seems not to hear me, lost in pain,
　Medicine, confusion
That has become her daily fare.

I shouldn't take the time; other patients wait,
　But I kneel beside her, facing the light,
Place my cheek near hers to direct her gaze:
　"Look, Louise," I repeat, "the deer are eating
　Blackberries."

After a moment I sense a response. "Deer,"
　She whispers. Then, "Two," she says
And I know she can see them.

They are eating quickly, rippling tan haunches
    To trouble the flies, feasting on the most accessible
    Fruit, oblivious to us watching.

All day she speaks of the deer. And the next day.
    For the last two weeks of her life
She talks of nothing else
    Her dry lips moving as though enjoying
        Blackberries.

As a hospice nurse, I have worked in a variety of settings. Although this patient was very confused, seeing the gentle animals outside her window helped make her final days, and even her death, peaceful and beautiful.

The Forgotten World

ELIZABETH COHEN

Once, this was a sparse planet,
a few scattered daffodils,
a lake of stars.
But it grew.

Things were piling on:
People were standing in crowds
without names.
There were oceans, continents,
the instructions for the tape recorder,
the way to retrieve messages from the phone machine,
gadgets to make ice.

And then the alphabet came,
numbers, Roman and Arabic,
the way to the bathroom at Riverview Manor,
the purpose of a fork.

And last of all came the basic things,
the way to swallow, to stand.
Anything you might desire is here,
on this planet, all these sad and lost things.

They each have their story.
They could howl like lost dogs,
They could sing,
and if they did,
if they sang and sang and sang,
they might sing back the memories
of a few small things, like birds
that come back in the spring.
But then those too would have to migrate.

I took care of my father, who died of Alzheimer's disease, for several years at the end of his life. During that time I watched him forgetting things—ranging from his whereabouts to his own name—which was so sad. But then I started to look at it differently. Maybe the things he was forgetting were simply going somewhere else. Not lost, but traveling to another planet, where all forgotten things go to wait for the person who knew them. It was comforting to think of it this way. That somewhere, somehow, all his memories were preserved and that now he has been reunited with them.

Magnolias

MARGOT WIZANSKY

They have moved here to die;
do not speak of slow interment.
They could lose a day hunting

a piece of paper. They pluck
at themselves in the manner of the senile.
Their backs round more and more.

Outside, late magnolias, extravagant
as ball gowns, blacken in sweet decay.
No one notices this quick birth and death.

And memory is an exhalation. They have given up
even each other's names—friends of their waning,
friends of their splintering.

None of them wants the startle of loud noise
or color, spice in their food, heartbreak or grief—
too late for the heavy perfume of the blossom.

"Magnolias" was written after a visit to my mother, who moved to a senior "village" after my stepfather's death. How difficult it must be to make new friends when one needs all one's energy to remember the details of life.

Time with the Dying

LINDA ALEXANDER

What shines about the dying?
Like a yellow petal backlit
by summer. The white of cold
pressed paper behind azure.

If you sit beside them long
enough. Hold a water glass
with a straw they can barely
sip through. You will know.

If you turn their pillow or put
on another blanket. Wait
patiently. They search for
a word to utter, *thank you.*

The way everything from this
world is still precious to them.
Every kindness a tender new
sun they want to hand you.

To watch a loved one dying, as I did my father, seems so difficult to the inexperi-enced; onlookers comment about the kindness of the caretaker. Yet if we observe more deeply, the dying teach us about the preciousness of things we take for granted: a glass of water, a cool pillow, one more moment with a loved one. It is the dying who are utterly kind to us, returning back to us everything of this world with their simple, silent gratitude.

Great Egrets

THEODORE DEPPE

Foghorns sound over brilliant, clear waters,
and egrets—as if unwilling to leave—drag their legs
above the harbor. A train glints along Stonington's

far shore but doesn't stop here anymore. Returning
to a house that's empty while my wife visits her sister,
I see an old woman—a neighbor I've never met—

standing confused, a grey stillness on Water Street.
No traffic, at least, but she's poised out there, staring at me.
At last, she says that a burglar's in her house.

I offer to call police, but she says, *That might be
embarrassing—they'll probably find the place empty
again.* Eighty-six, out walking her dog for five minutes

and already she fears going home. Dirty bare feet
sheathed in sneakers, white hair plumed in wind.
We check both chaotic floors: no one's

in the book-constricted rooms though it's easy to see
why she might think someone's ransacked
this house: sweaters and peacock scarves

strewn on Persian rugs, overturned whisky glasses,
but no sign of a prowler, no evidence
of her son's girlfriend *who sometimes comes*

and messes my sheets while I'm out.
She lights a cigarette, lights mine, talks with a stranger
until her voice is calm.

Eighty-six: Marie's the same age as my wife's mother was
when the phone call came. I made coffee
before waking Annie, then left it in the kitchen,

climbed into bed and held her as she
startled into my arms—*What's wrong. Something's*
wrong! I don't know any good way to break such news.

Tonight, when I said good-bye a second time, Marie asked,
What season is it? Not what day or what year but what season.
Her little poodle slept in the windowsill.

I said it was fall, and asked had she seen the egrets?
Oh, she said, *if it's fall your egrets will be leaving soon.*
When they want to go, you know, all you can do is let them go.

"Great Egrets" was written during a year's residency in the James Merrill House in
Stonington, Connecticut. I found that memory was one of the important subjects
in the book of poems I was writing while I was there. Memory is so vulnerable, so
often unreliable, so precious.

XI.
Winter Solstice

Winter Solstice

ELLEN KIRVIN DUDIS

Days are getting shorter, your mother's light
as well. She doesn't understand the waning.
This morning finds us once again explaining.
But it's so dark she says. And then at night,
It's dark so early. Each time we recite
the seasons, winter losing, summer gaining,
it feels as though the universe is ours
—but not the space of habit still remaining
when she says *you're right* again, *you're right,*
her eyes gone vacant as collapsing stars.
Still, we insist our universe be hers.
But what's the use? The sun sets earlier
and earlier. The universe devours
dying light. It's dark. All our winters are.

*My husband's mother is now fading into senility. Our experience with my mother
has taught us a little about coping with our frustration, but the instinctive reaction
to insist she understand the nature of things, to somehow will her to comprehend
again, still rises all too often.*

Where We Have Come

SUSAN LUDVIGSON

1. The Solace of Poems

To discover them
is to link with the unbroken
griefs we name and rename.

The death, by degrees,
of a mother
is a kind of death
of self.

Without a mirror
I see my face,
her mouth pinched;
know, from the inside,
fingers tapping the table,
an almost demure
drop of the head.

This is part of it.

But to see loss
black on white
is to be comforted
a moment
in the early hours,
not left alone
to mourn a mind
dropping its history
like Gretel's bread,
birds swooping behind.

2. After the Latest Descent

Slow motion
through the death
that is not
death enough,
room after room
locking, locked, where
creatures caught inside
scratch at windows,
at the light
under doors.

The keys turn, by contrast,
quietly. Something determined
slips down the halls,
listening, as children disappear
in the airless chambers,
then husbands, Christmas
dinners, faces
in frames

until only the snake brain
remains in the stubborn,
irrelevant body.

She is halfway there.
This is minor preparation.

3. What Does It Matter

that another old woman goes,
mind first, her words
become less lovely
than whirs of wings at night
in the disturbed bamboo,
a startled rapping against leaves
that takes the heart.

4. Where We Have Come

Walking the same
green path, day
after day, we watched a duck
drop an egg, later
ducklings like a yellow fan
on the red-brown water.
This is where we sat,
where I tried to teach us
concentration.

She is moving toward
peace—the first time
in her life, now,
as her brain knots
its fine yarns.
How can it be? At the same time
that something releases,
something like god
enters her. Her laugh
is girlish, full
of delight.

Death is still
a stranger, but
he carries lilacs.

*"Where We Have Come" was written during a period after we'd placed my mother
in an assisted living facility in the town where my husband and I live in South
Carolina. She had spent her whole life in Wisconsin. I had been away from there,
and from her, for so long that I hadn't realized how much I still identified with
her. My grieving for her began then, as I watched her decline. I took her for walks
in a park, where I was foolish enough to think that we might practice meditation
sitting on a bench together. Needless to say, this was not possible, but I did see
her, on those walks, begin to be at peace and to take pleasure in small things—
birdsong, watching the ducks on the pond, even, amazingly, simple jokes that
depended on wordplay.*

Augury

KENITH SIMMONS

We read your breakfast tray like tea leaves:
Do you have a future?
Sodium levels 165:
Your body is shutting down.
Five days on a dextrose drip;
Sodium levels 135:
Perfectly normal,
And your veins are collapsing.
You hadn't taken food or drink in days.
You doze, eyes closed,
Eyes open, seeing nothing we can see.
We argue, splinters in our hearts,
Make awful choices on which we disagree.
Disconnected.
We disconnect you.
Disconnected, you
Eat breakfast:
Mashed waffles, pureed ham,
Suck maple syrup right from the spoon.
Magic pudding,
Miracle shake,
Miraculous:
Two hours straight,
Dozing and waking,
Chewing and chewing.
Smiling and not at nothing.
At us,
Your astonished family,
Giddy with your sheer presence
Among us again.
We want to read,

As if the half-empty plates
Were the entrails of birds,
Your future.

I wrote this poem in February 2005 as I watched my mother sleep. I had been asked by the family and her doctor to fly home immediately, since she had stopped eating and her death was imminent. The family was bitterly divided as to how to manage her end-of-life care. She died in August 2005.

Augury

JOEL A. MCCOLLOUGH

The cruelest month, foolsday,
and on my drive to the hospital
the jay in the puddled gutter bats
a blue halo around its smashed half,
and a thrasher hugs the double line,
one brown wing vaning every passage.

I meet my mother in the lobby,
her hand fluttering to her mouth.
"He's bleeding," she whispers.
In room 314 my grandfather falls,
arms spread as if to span a crucifix
or fly up from one.

They have cinched his wrists
to the bedrails because he's bound
to pluck out the IV and wires.
He lies swathed in snowy surplus,
linen lapped with a crimson sash,
Roman senator of the old Republic,
august, ashen, forecasting the assassin.

I was mistaken, one year and counting,
having divined all the wrong signs.
Today I feed him strawberry ice cream,
nesting the spoon in a pink beak
under the breezy clemency of trees,
sunshot, green-plumed and populous.
We cannot speak for singing.

"Augury" documents the hospitalization and the unlikely recovery of my grand-father, Homer Earl Durham, during his battle with Alzheimer's. I had prepared myself for the worst outcome. Everything I saw seemed to foretell our loss.

Reprieve

PAULANN PETERSEN

Through the phone a woman's voice asks
if I am my name, and when I answer *yes,*
tells me she'll put my mother on the line.
A crazy lightning sheers through my pulse
as I say *my mother?* not thinking of
little miracles, windows of clarity—
surely not that unheard of—
when the random notes of Alzheimer's
might suddenly form a pure chord,
sweet sound of my mother saying
I don't want to be any bother,
but come get me, I need to go home.
But quickly: the woman's confusion in the face
of my confusion, her stumbled apology.
She doesn't usually work this part of the floor,
she got mixed up, but my mom's just fine, actually
she's placing a call for my mother's roommate
and grabbed the wrong name and number,
oh dear, she can see how the call would be a shock
and she's sorry, really sorry, but my mother
is fine, doing just fine.
          Hanging up,
I'm stunned, wishing I'd said without hesitation
Yes, put her on, wanting to believe
that with faith, whole and unwavering,
I'd have heard my mother—
her voice finding something on her mind,
maybe slow and faltering, but yes, just fine—
heard her speak to me one more time.

My mother lived her last four years as the sole patient in a caregiver's home. To give the caregiver a much-needed break from round-the-clock responsibilities, hospice would occasionally arrange for my mother to spend a few days in a hospital facility.

The Inland Sea

DAVID MASON

All the little fears have schooled and darted
out to the hallway's regulated shoals,
the numbered rooms, the doors with coded locks
in case of trouble. Here the patients drift,
fish-jawed in their medicated stupors.

Mouthing dialects that no one understands,
their faces float up and their guileless eyes
look out at us, their brains a weedy bed
of plaques and tangles. They will leave us trapped
inside the real and comprehensible—

or leave us, anyway, to walk the hall
and try the door out to the tiny terrace
with its trellis like a cage or crab pot.
We find them there bewildered by the bars
and turn them back into the inland sea.

Their dignity another universe
might honor more than we do, seeing souls
where we see bodies failing into death.
Some fear is always lurking in the shadows,
some violence they can't explain. Drowned children,

they hold hands in plausible innocence,
as if in mastery of discipline,
both past and future utterly dissolved.
Their beauty terrifies us, so we think
it like no beauty we have ever known

and leave them for the ordinary shore.

The last time I saw my father alive he was adrift in the home, but as if some part of his old personality survived, he seemed to be looking for a way to escape. As I watched the heavily medicated patients move in the halls of that building north of Seattle, it suddenly seemed to me that my horror at their condition was misplaced, that in some weird way they were even beautiful, or that my notion of beauty would have to be adjusted to make room for what these people had become.

The Withering of Their State

JUDY KRONENFELD

> And all that believed were together, and had all things common.
>   ACTS 2:44

In the end they lose all
their chains and ghost and swirl
by each other in the closed
bubble of the "reminiscence"
wing like flakes of snow
in an upended souvenir globe.

In the end they wander in
the deserts of each other's
synonymous small rooms,
their possessions winnowed
like so much chaff in a chill
breeze, sold by
beleaguered daughters, parted
to Goodwill— the leavings squeezed
in with the new twin bed: one table,
one uneasy chair, the old TV
they have forgotten how to turn on.

And in the end no one among them
lacks, for if one sits shivering
on the toilet, where the attendant
has deposited him, dreaming and
losing a dream of dry warmth
like a distant bell, the groaning wardrobe
of his roommate may yet open unto him.

And in the end the scales fall
from their eyes, and they fall asleep
in each other's chairs, and thine
is mine, and now is then, and mildly,
with the most gracious of *oh?*s,
they allow themselves to be
removed, guided away by their pliant
elbows, by those who still live
in the bordered world.

The seed for this poem was planted when I told a friend how my father's belong-
ings kept disappearing in his facility's euphemistically named dementia wing. She
said, "And we never were communists!" Eventually, the Bible, Marx, and other
registers of language combined to mourn, protest, imagine accepting the loss of
the personal, personhood, the person.

Letting Go

JOAN I. SIEGEL

All day
the day before he died
my father squeezed my hand
the way a child holds on tight
when he leaves home for the first time.

What was he seeing with his eyes shut?

Was he watching himself go out for the morning paper
and suddenly the street dropped off into nothing
like the edge of a map and someone erased the street
back to his house?

Was he looking inside the dark room of his brain
to find it had been ransacked by thugs
who had yanked the fixtures from the ceiling
ripped the pictures off the wall?

The next day he let go—
gathering courage like a boy
at the edge of a dark, cold lake:
sucking air and diving in at last
for the first time.

I wrote my way through grief of my father's illness and death. I always wondered what he saw behind his eyes. I like to think that he heard me speaking to him, felt me holding his hand. The day before he died, he knew he had to let go and was saying good-bye.

XII.
Still Life

His Funeral

JEFF WORLEY

My father was finally unconfused,
the noose of Alzheimer's snapped.
Around him the malodorous roses
and long shafts of lilies.

I squeezed his shoulder, patted it
like the flank of a favorite dog.
I knew this was a dumb, sentimental
gesture. I didn't care.

My sister said—the whole room listening—
that our father had gone now
to a better place. The funeral home
claque nodded like breeze-bent stalks.

I wished for a long moment my sister
was right, but then two men came
and closed the light from him.
His new roof screwed tightly down,

I could still hear him say, *A better place,
Joyce? Show me the evidence.* The organ
shook down dust from the oak beams.
Joyce sang loudly along on the first hymn
with the few people who'd come. In my head
I sang "Don't Fence Me In." Dad told me
he'd hummed this when the gates
of Stalag XI-B were flung open,
and he hobbled out on makeshift crutches.
He was headed back to Kansas, its glorious
dullness and flatness, bars of sunshine

in his father's field, the amazing grace
of wheat and wheat and wheat.

*As a poet, I was happy to be able to get my father back to Kansas—he was born
and raised in Abilene. And I was very pleased that this poem won* Atlanta Review's
international poetry competition in 2002.

Death Picks Up My Aunt, Huldah Bell

KAKE HUCK

Absence is always too soon for someone.
Standing at the door, discussing
fat peonies on the porch or leftovers
boxed to carry home, the body remains
among the things it knew. While there outside,
already in the car, tired of making small talk,
the mind is waiting, leaning on the horn.

This lengthy last discussion disturbs
those who remain behind, still busy
with the party. "Just go or stay,"
we whisper to each other, wink-grimacing
our disapproval. Such fragmentation
disrupts our practiced tales of war
and marriage told with brandy
and that second piece of cake.

I lived with my dad's sister, Huldah Bell, my first year in college. She introduced me to my future life partner and was a major support my next thirteen years. After I left for graduate school, we kept in touch. On one return I noticed she was forgetting simple words. The problem grew worse, and finally a group of friends and siblings helped her move into a care facility. Finally, bereft of sense, she was moved to a hospital nursing home where she was an empty vessel, caved in, her eyes sometimes bright but usually vacant. Then she died. Her decay haunts me as I notice myself growing more forgetful.

A Woodpecker Taps

PAMELA MILLER NESS

First day
of the year you did not
live to see
foothills shrouded
lightly in fog.

Winter rain:
waiting at the station
for the tram
that goes where you
no longer are.

These trees
you photographed . . .
Why
do I see only
empty branches?

So warm
this winter of your death;
beneath
our chestnut tree
a clump of snowdrops.

Cold rain
this first day of spring;
I discard
can after can of old paint,
the plaid shirt you never wore.

Soft rain
high above the path
we walked
a woodpecker taps
and taps again.

Whitman wrote:
Look for me under
your boot soles.
And I do.
And you are.

This is the fourth part of a tanka sequence written over a period of six years, detailing two journeys: my father's journey into Alzheimer's disease and my journey as daughter, caregiver, and translator of our experience into words. "A Woodpecker Taps" was written during the year after my father's death.

Still Life

ELLEN KIRVIN DUDIS

My mother's brain floats in a jar
on its way to Johns Hopkins. Doctors there
will try to find out why and when and where
so much went missing.

They will cut deeper and deeper
into the strange lifeless interior,
sifting the ruined amphitheater
of the lost city

cell by cell, questioning the blur
they bring to light. Tell us. How could she obscure
herself to death? Look—I send a picture—
this was my mother!

No one else will ever fill a jar
with purple loosestrife and give it the flair
she, too, was artlessly as unaware
of as the flowers.

The Alzheimer's research unit at Johns Hopkins asked me for a brief biography of my mother. In giving them a thumbnail "life story," I suddenly realized how little the facts convey and wanted these strangers to appreciate the person my mother was—which was coming back to me in a flood of regrets.

Goodwill

MARIE BAHLKE

He drops your old self
on the concrete floor.
"Receipt, lady?"
I gaze at this untidiness—
one Harris tweed sleeve
pledging allegiance.
A sleeve that does tricks.
What is that worth?
The tan corduroy.
Perfect for travel
you told me on the bus
to Gubbio. Your coat
of many pockets, you'd laugh,
playing Joseph all over
Europe. The "lecherous
old man coat" you'd
never put on.
Full value for that?
Buried under all,
Scottish caps, Norwegian
hat like that King's.
Red-cheeked, you claimed
it powered your skis
up Kellogg Forest hills.
"Receipt, lady?"
For this travelogue?
This messy heap
about to reshape itself
while you sit where
you are, quiet,
a little lunch

left on your lip,
belt buckled in the back.

No longer able to face that half a closet of lonely clothes, I chose November's bitter-
est day to lay them carefully on the car's backseat and then drive down the alley
past garbage cans and trash containers to Goodwill's pick-up door.

Lane Change

PAULANN PETERSEN

A snapshot glance over my shoulder,
and I make my move, quick, thinking
how easy, how simple to
not see, to hit, be hit: the blindside
slash of metal, of glass,
my flesh driven back into the sharp
of my own teeth and bones.
Smashed just like that,
and maybe not even a stop

for pain. Maybe my mind
plucks me away from my done-for
body, lets me think I live on,
still driving the now gone-to-scrap car
onto the arc of bridge that each day routes me
home. Driving up, over the river's sheen,
cresting above midflow, then down
onto the other side and off, until it's all
a pure coast.

Maybe my mother's last years
were such a thing. Those motionless,
voiceless days, not days or nights
at all, not a senseless dragging
of flesh, not some nightmare sleep
that kept her awake enough
to chew, to swallow,
her bowels and bladder emptied
by tubes. Not that, but just
her behind the wheel,
some sun easing through the windshield,

dust whispered along the dash,
a tune she likes on the radio,
little hum harboring somewhere
in her throat. Here comes the approach
to the bridge, and another driver stops
long enough to let her into the line
of crossing cars. A wave of thanks,

then a slow climb to the part
she likes best, at the bridge's crest.
There she can glimpse a mountain's point
and a river's mirror length,
the part that could just as well last forever
if anyone bothered to ask her.
Up and over the narrow span—that one drive
she could do in her sleep,
the easy one, home.

My mother spent the last two years of her life reduced to a vegetative state by Alzheimer's. During that time, I dreamed and fervently hoped that—deep within herself—she was living a rich, sweet life.

My Father Calls

GARY THOMPSON

My father calls from wherever
he's dead to ask about things
in his hesitant telephone voice
that can't quite believe
he's connected to me.

He's worried about Mother,
her evening shower, the outside care
I've arranged, the chocolates
she'd devour if I let her.
He's alive with advice, excited.

It's a common dream—
sons being summoned
by dead fathers—how the boy
in Michigan hid
when his just dead grandfather

returned for their bedtime
story and goodnight kiss.
And years later, when there was only
numb darkness and a gun
and a bed lamp at his side, how that

reminded him to live.

Our family lived with my mother's Alzheimer's for fifteen years, and when my father died, I took over responsibility for her care. Her last three years here were difficult, yes, but strangely poignant too, even joyous. Now I think of it as the haunting disease—literally for those it strikes, and figuratively for those of us who care for and love them.

Dreaming My Mother in the Bone Church, Kostnice

SUSAN LUDVIGSON

Five years after her death,
I take her hand, lead her
onto a dance floor.

A door opens, a breeze flits through,
and the chandelier sings,
throat bones dangling
crystal, finger bones
keeping time.

Ringed with skulls,
woven white wrists
warp and woof a loose
call to mass
note by clicking note.

Death is the mother of beauty,
we've been told, and here,
a few miles from Prague,
the woodcarver Frantisek Rindt,
commissioned by monks
to transform the remains
of 40,000 dead
into "pleasing arrangements," did.

For this grace,
her body doesn't need
what was once her mind.
We glide near

the coat of arms bones
studded with knuckles
rosaries of knuckles
vases and crosses, chalice
and pyramid of hip bones.
In falling light,
fibias swirl.

Her blue skirt flares
as she twirls. We skim

through arches and doorways
toward fleur-de-lys bones,
bones of the toes making roses.

As the sun comes up slowly
in South Carolina, in March,
I wake to my life
in a strange contentment.

Is there anything left to wish for?

*"Dreaming My Mother in the Bone Church, Kostnice" came out of a dream that
ended with my mother and me dancing together. I woke up feeling intensely happy.
In the dream, the setting wasn't Kostnice, but I had been reading about that place,
which seemed exactly right for this poem.*

Contributors

Ჯ

LINDA ALEXANDER, a native Floridian, is an artist, writer, and teacher She has written and illustrated over a dozen children's books. Her poetry, influenced by the natural world and her indigenous heritage, has been published in anthologies and journals and won her several awards, including the Taos Summer Writers' Conference Merit Scholarship for poetry and the Writer's Voice Hibiscus Award for her chapbook *Natural Elements*.

GILBERT ALLEN has lived in Travelers Rest, South Carolina, with his wife, Barbara, since 1977. He teaches at Furman University. His collections of poems are *In Everything, Second Chances, Commandments at Eleven,* and *Driving to Distraction,* which was featured on Garrison Keillor's *The Writer's Almanac.* In 2005, he coedited *A Millennial Sampler of South Carolina Poetry.* His chapbook *Body Parts* was published by the South Carolina Poetry Initiative in 2007.

JANE ALYNN is the author of the collection of poems *Threads & Dust* (Finishing Line Press, 2005). Her poems have been published in numerous journals, including *The Pacific Review, Quercus Review, Snowy Egret,* and *Switched-on Gutenberg.* In 2004 she won a William Stafford Award from the Washington Poets Association.

ARLENE ANG lives in Venice, Italy, where she coedits the Italian edition of *Niederngasse.* Her poetry has been published in *Envoi, Orbis, The Pedestal, Rattle, Smiths Knoll,* and *Poetry Ireland.* Her first full collection of poetry, *The Desecration of Doves,* is available online.

JUDITH ARCANA's most recent book is the poetry collection *What if your mother;* among her prose books is *Grace Paley's Life Stories: A Literary Biography.* Her work has appeared recently in print and online in *5AM, The Persimmon Tree, White Ink, Bridges, Umbrella, ARM Journal,* and *Passager;* more is forthcoming in journals and anthologies.

E. A. AXELBERG's poems have appeared in *Cumberland Poetry Review, North Dakota Quarterly, The Antigonish Review,* and *Hidden Oak Poetry Journal.* She is a former copy editor for *The Atlanta Journal-Constitution* and has articles published in *Atlanta Magazine.* Her father passed away after struggling with dementia for several years.

LANA HECHTMAN AYERS is a manuscript consultant, a workshop facilitator, poetry editor of *Crab Creek Review,* and publisher of the *Concrete Wolf Poetry Chapbook Series* and the *Late Blooms Poetry Postcard Series.* She is the author of two collections, *Chicken Farmer I Still Love You* (D-N Publishing) and *Dance From Inside Her Bones* (Snake Nation Press). Visit her website to read more of her work.

MARIE BAHLKE began writing for solace and sustenance during her husband's seven-year struggle with Alzheimer's disease. Her poetry collection *One Oar* won first place in the poetry category of Writer's Digest 12th Annual International Self-Published Book Awards.

MARY BARRETT is a freelance writer who writes for the *Berkeley Daily Planet,* has published several poems in literary magazines, and is working on a collection of stories about teaching. She just retired after thirty-five years of teaching in the Berkeley, California, public schools.

JUDITH BARRINGTON is the author of three volumes of poetry: *Horses and the Human Soul* (2004), *History and Geography* (1989), and *Trying to Be an Honest Woman* (1985). Her most recent publication is a chapbook of poems: *Postcard from the Bottom of the Sea* (2008). Her *Lifesaving: A Memoir* won the 2001 Lambda Book Award and was a finalist for the PEN/Martha Albrand Award for the Art of the Memoir.

RICHARD BEBAN is a Los Angeles–based poet whose first book, *What the Heart Weighs,* was published by Red Hen Press in late 2004. His second book, *Young Girl Eating a Bird,* was published by Red Hen in 2006.

DAN BELLM lives in San Francisco and has published three books of poetry: *One Hand on the Wheel* (Heyday Books, 2003), *Buried Treasure* (Cleveland State University, 1999), and *Practice* (Sixteen Rivers Press, 2008). His poems and translations from Spanish have appeared in *Poetry, Ploughshares, The Threepenny Review, The Village Voice,* and other journals and anthologies.

KATE BERNADETTE BENEDICT is the author of the poetry collection *Here from Away* (CustomWords) and the editor of *Umbrella,* an online poetry journal.

BRUCE BERGER's poems have appeared in *Poetry, Barron's,* and *Orion* and have been collected in *Facing the Music.* His prose works include *The Telling Distance,* winner of the Western States Book Award. His recent *Oasis of Stone* won the *ForeWord* Silver Award. As a relief from words, he plays benefit classical piano concerts in Mexico.

MARION BOYER teaches at Kalamazoo Valley Community College. Finishing Line Press published her poetry chapbook, *Green,* in November 2003. Her poetry has appeared most recently in *Atlanta Review's 10th Anniversary Anthology, The Spoon River Poetry Review, Midwest Quarterly, Heliotrope, Permafrost, Rhino,* and *The MacGuffin.*

CATHLEEN CALBERT is the author of three books of poetry: *Lessons in Space* (University of Florida Press, 1997), *Bad Judgment* (Sarabande Books, 1999), and *Sleeping with a Famous Poet* (CustomWords, 2007). Her awards include *The Nation* Discovery Award, and a Pushcart Prize. She holds the Tucker Thorp Professorship at Rhode Island College, where she directs the creative writing program.

JOANNE M. CLARKSON changed careers after twenty years of working as a professional librarian and became a registered nurse, working in hospice. Next to family, poetry has always been her greatest love. She has published three books of poems, including *Pacing the Moon* (Chantry Press) and *Crossing without Daughters* (March Street Press).

SHEBANA COELHO is a writer and producer of documentaries for radio and television. She received a 2004 Fiction Fellowship from the New York Foundation for the Arts (NYFA) and is working on a short story collection and a novel. She was born in Bombay, India, and currently lives in New York.

ELIZABETH COHEN is a reporter for the *Press & Sun Bulletin* in Binghamton, New York. Her memoir, *The House on Beartown Road: A Memoir of Learning and Forgetting*, published by Random House in 2003 (now in paperback as *The Family on Beartown Road: A Memoir of Love and Courage*), is a chronicle of the year she spent caring for her father, who had Alzheimer's disease, and her infant daughter in a remote farmhouse in upstate New York.

ALLAN DOUGLASS COLEMAN writes poetry, fiction, and creative nonfiction; makes music and photographs; and produces various other forms of visual art. Under the pen name A. D. Coleman, he is an internationally published critic, historian, and curator of photography. His first collection of poetry and prose poetry, *Spine*, appeared in 2000; the second, *Like Father Like Son*, a collaboration with the poet Earl Coleman, came out in 2007.

NINA CORWIN, a Chicago social worker, is the author of *Conversations with Friendly Demons and Tainted Saints* (Puddin'head Press, 1999) and coeditor of *Inhabiting the Body: A Collection of Poetry and Art by Women* (Moon Journal Press, 2002). Her published work appears in the anthologies *Visiting Frost* (University of Iowa Press, 2005) and *Poetic Voices Without Borders* (Gival Press) and various literary journals. She has received awards from the Illinois Arts Council and the Illinois State Poetry Society.

RACHEL DACUS has three poetry collections, *Another Circle of Delight*, *Femme au chapeau*, and *Earth Lessons*. Her poetry CDs are *A God You Can Dance* and *Singing in the Pandaleshwar Caves*. She serves as contributing poetry editor for *Umbrella* and as a staff member of the *Alsop Review*. More of her work can be read online.

CAROLYN DAHL's poems have been published in *Sojourn*, *TimeSlice*, *Suddenly*, *Echoes for a New Room*, *Natural Impressions*, *The Texas Poetry Calendars*, the

2008 Women Artists Datebook, and *The Weight of Addition Anthology.* She was a finalist award winner in the PEN Texas competition and has received grants from the Texas Commission for the Arts. She is currently working on a book of memoir essays.

NANCY DAHLBERG is on the board of PoetsWest and is membership chair of Washington Poets Association. Her poems have been published in journals such as *Shenandoah, Calyx, Stringtown, Northwest Review,* and *Chrysanthemum,* as well as in the anthology *Limbs of the Pine, Peaks of the Range.* She was a finalist in the 2005–6 Seattle Poet Populist competition.

BRIAN DALDORPH teaches at the University of Kansas, Lawrence. He edits *Coal City Review.* His most recent book of poetry is *Senegal Blues* (219 Press, 2003), and he has a new book coming out: *From the Inside Out: Sonnets* (Woodley Press, 2008). He has taught in England, Senegal, Zambia, and Japan.

JOHN DAVIS teaches high school and plays in the rock 'n' roll band Never Been To Utah. He has published poetry in *Beloit Poetry Journal, The Laurel Review, Passages North, Poetry Northwest,* and *The Seattle Review.* His chapbook, *The Reservist,* appears from Pudding House Press.

LORENE DELANY-ULLMAN is a native Californian who received her MFA from the University of California, Irvine, in June 2003. She was the managing editor for volume 12 of *Faultline,* UC Irvine's literary journal. She is also one of the founding members of the *Casa Romantica* Poetry Reading Series, which is a committee of local southern California writers who organize monthly poetry readings in south Orange County.

THEODORE DEPPE is the author of four collections of poems, most recently *Cape Clear: New and Selected Poems.* He is writer-in-residence at Phillips Academy in Andover, Massachusetts, and teaches in the Stonecoast MFA program. His work has been recognized with NEA grants and a Pushcart Prize.

ALICE DERRY has three collections of poems. The most recent, *Strangers to Their Courage,* from Louisiana State University Press (2001), was a finalist for the Washington Book Award. She teaches at Peninsula College in Port Angeles, Washington, where she is codirector of the Foothills Writers' Series.

ELLEN DUDIS lives on Maryland's eastern shore. She has published poems in many national journals and newspapers. Her manuscript, "Gratitudes," continues to look for a publisher.

ELIZABETH FARRELL's poems have appeared in the anthology *Proposing on the Brooklyn Bridge, Animus, Calliope, The Onset Review, New Bedford Magazine,* and many other publications. She has worked as an advertising copywriter and been writer-in-residence in several schools in southeastern Massachusetts.

LINDA ANNAS FERGUSON is the author of four collections of poetry, most recently *Bird Missing from One Shoulder* (WordTech Editions, 2007). She was the 2005 Poetry Fellow for the South Carolina Arts Commission and served as the

2003–4 poet-in-residence for the Gibbes Museum of Art in Charleston, South Carolina. A recipient of the poetry fellowship of the South Carolina Academy of Authors, she was recently elected to the Academy's Board of Governors.

TESS GALLAGHER's caregiving of her mother spanned nearly seventeen years, during which her mother suffered a stroke and eventually entered dementia and Alzheimer's. She recognizes this period as one of the strongest, most formative of her life. She is a poet, fiction writer, essayist, screenplay writer, and translator. Her poetry collections include *Moon Crossing Bridge, Amplitude: New and Selected Poems,* and, most recently, *Dear Ghosts,* all of which are available from Graywolf Press. She lives in Port Angeles, Washington.

MADELYN GARNER has long served Colorado students as a teacher and administrator. An ardent supporter of the arts, she has been the recipient of numerous honors, including the Governor's Award for Excellence in the Arts and Humanities. Recently, the University of New Mexico recognized her writing with a D. H. Lawrence Fellowship. Her award-winning poems have appeared in *MARGIE, CALYX, Harpur Palate, Georgetown Review,* and *Water-Stone Review.*

ARTHUR GINSBERG is a neurologist and poet based in Seattle. He has published work in many poetry and medical journals. His work appears in the anthology *Blood and Bone* from University of Iowa Press, and his book, *Walking the Panther,* was published by Northwoods Press in 1984. He was awarded the William Stafford prize in 2003 by the Washington Poets Association.

DIANE PORTER GOFF is a writer and photographer who lives and works in the mountains of Virginia. Her work has appeared in many publications, among them *The Sun Magazine, We'Moon Calendar* books, and *Southern Distinctions Magazine.* She has just completed a memoir, "Riding the Elephant, An Alzheimer's Journey."

JOSEPH GREEN lives in Longview, Washington, where he has taught English at Lower Columbia College for the last twenty-two years. A chapbook of his poems, *The End of Forgiveness,* is available from Floating Bridge Press.

JOHN GREY is an Australian-born poet, playwright, and musician, who has been a U.S. resident since the late 1970s. His latest book is *What Else Is There* from Main Street Rag. His work has appeared recently in *Hubbub, South Carolina Review,* and *Journal of the American Medical Association.*

ROB HARDY's poetry chapbook *The Collecting Jar* won the 2004 Grayson Books Poetry Chapbook Competition. He has been a stay-at-home father, worked as a substitute teacher, written scripts for Garrison Keillor, taught Latin to Catholic seminarians, and led a writing group for secular homeschoolers.

JAN HARRINGTON has lived near Geneva, Switzerland, for eight years. Her poems have appeared in literary journals in Europe. She travels often to the United States to help care for her father.

PENNY HARTER's latest book of poems is *The Night Marsh.* She has received fellowships from the New Jersey State Arts Council and the Dodge Foundation and a prize from the Poetry Society of America. Her poems in *American Nature Writing 2002* won the William O. Douglas Nature Writing Award.

ESTHER ALTSHUL HELFGOTT writes in Seattle, Washington. Her most recent publications include *Analytic Entrapment* (*American Imago*) and *Irena Klepfisz, Loss and the Poetry of Exile* (*Journal of Poetry Therapy*). She teaches writing and cares for her husband, Abe, a retired pathologist, who now has Alzheimer's.

CHRISTINE HIGGINS, a McDowell Colony Fellow and a graduate of the Writing Seminars, is the recipient of a Maryland State Arts Council Award. Her poems have appeared in several journals, including *Pequod, Lullwater Review, Passager, Eleventh Muse,* and *America.*

EDWARD HIRSCH has published six books of poems, including *Wild Gratitude* (1986), which won the National Book Critics Circle Award, and *Lay Back the Darkness* (2003). He has also published four prose books, including *How to Read a Poem,* a national bestseller, and *Poet's Choice* (2006). He is president of the Guggenheim Foundation.

KAKE HUCK has published in small journals such as *Alehouse, Ekphrasis, Freshwater, Harpur Palate, The High Desert Journal,* and others. Her work is included in two anthologies, *Women's Encounters with the Mental Health Establishment* and *Regrets Only.* The poem included in this volume won the 2K3 Poetry Award from the Peralta Press, where it was first printed. The IRS considers her poetry a hobby, not work.

HOLLY J. HUGHES's chapbook *Boxing the Compass* won the 2007 Floating Bridge Press chapbook award. Her poems have appeared in various literary magazines and several anthologies, most recently *Dancing with Joy: 99 Poems* (Random House). A graduate of the Rainier Writing Workshop MFA program, she co-directs the Convergence Writers Series at Edmonds Community College.

M. J. IUPPA lives on a small farm near the shore of Lake Ontario. Her poems have appeared in *Tar River Poetry, miller's pond, Iconoclast, The Modern Review* (Canada), *Coffee House* (UK), *Flint Hills Review, Canter Collected, Rosebud, HazMat Review, The Comstock Review, Tar Wolf Review,* and *Pearl.* She has three chapbooks and a full-length collection, *Night Traveler* (Foothills Publishing, 2003), and is the writer-in-residence and director of the arts minor program at St. John Fisher College.

RICK KEMPA lives in Rock Springs, Wyoming, where he directs the honors program at Western Wyoming College. "Prayer for My Mother" is part of the collection *Nothing Between Us Now But Love,* which recounts his mother's struggle with Alzheimer's. Other poems and essays of his on this theme can be found in *Healing Muse, Ars Medica, Confrontation,* and *Conte Online.*

CLAIRE KEYES has published reviews and poems in *The Women's Review of Books, The Georgia Review, Zone3,* and *Blueline,* among others. She won first prize in the Beullah Rose Poetry Contest, sponsored by *Smartish Pace,* and the Robert Penn Warren Award (First Prize) from New England Writers. Her chapbook

Rising and Falling won the Foothills Poetry Chapbook Competition. She lives in Marblehead, Massachusetts, and teaches in the Lifelong Learning Program at Salem State College.

PERSIS KNOBBE has written short fiction for *American Fiction* (vol. 3), *An Inn Near Kyoto* (a travel collection), and *Marlboro Review.* Her short story, "Here I Am," provided the title for a collection from the Jewish Publication Society that won an Oakland PEN award. She writes periodically for the *San Francisco Chronicle* about her husband's journey through Alzheimer's.

JUDY KRONENFELD's second full-length collection of poetry *Light Lowering in Diminished Sevenths* won the 2007 Litchfield Review Book Award in poetry and will be published in 2008 by the Litchfield Review Press. She has published poetry in numerous print and online journals. She is also the author of a critical study, *King Lear and the Naked Truth* (Duke, 1998). She teaches in the creative writing department at University of California, Riverside.

SARAH LEAVITT regularly contributes writing and comics to *Geist* magazine and writes a monthly column for *Xtra West,* Vancouver's lesbian and gay newspaper. She has created short documentaries for CBC Radio, and her articles have appeared in the *Globe and Mail* and *Vancouver Review,* as well as a number of anthologies. She is working on a graphic memoir about her mother dying of Alzheimer's. Sarah's drawing and writing can be seen online.

NANCY TUPPER LING is the 2005 Grand Prize winner for *Writer's Digest*'s annual competition. Her poetry received second place in the Pacific Northwest Writers Association's annual contest. Her publication credits include *Potomac Review, Mid-American Poetry Review, Flyway,* and *Rambunctious Review.* She resides in Walpole, Massachusetts, with her husband and two daughters.

SYBIL LOCKHART writes and edits science and creative nonfiction In Berkeley, California. Her "Mama in the Middle" columns on caregiving and parenting can be found in *Literary Mama Magazine* online. Her book *Early Stages: A Biologist's Tale of Mothering and Daughtering* is forthcoming (Touchstone/ Simon & Schuster, 2009).

SUSAN LUDVIGSON is professor of English at Winthrop University. Her published books include seven titles from Louisiana State University Press, most recently *Escaping the House of Certainty* (2006). She is a recipient of fellowships from the Guggenheim, Rockefeller, Fulbright, and Witter Bynner foundations; from the National Endowment for the Arts; and from the North and South Carolina Arts Commissions. She has represented the United States at writers' meetings in France, Belgium, Canada, and Yugoslavia.

MELANIE MARTIN recently received her MFA in poetry from Southern Illinois University, Carbondale, and currently lives in California. She has poems published in *Southeast Review, The Chiron Review,* and *The Kali Guide.* She was the featured poet in *re)verb #2.*

DAVID MASON's books include *The Buried Houses, The Country I Remember, Arrivals,* and the verse novel *Ludlow.* His collection of essays *The Poetry of Life and the Life of Poetry* appeared in 2000, and he has coedited several textbooks and anthologies, including *Western Wind: An Introduction to Poetry, Twentieth Century American Poetry,* and *Rebel Angels: 25 Poets of the New Formalism.* A native of Washington state, Mason teaches at The Colorado College.

JOEL A. MCCOLLOUGH was a winner in the 2004 Piccolo Spoleto Short Fiction Open. His poetry has been nominated for a Pushcart Prize and has appeared in *Southern Poetry Review, Cumberland Poetry Review, Chattahoochee Review, Valparaiso Poetry Review, Poem, Illuminations,* and *A Millennial Sampler of South Carolina Poets* (Ninety-Six Press).

ETHNA MCKIERNAN's second book of poems is *The One Who Swears You Can't Start Over,* from Salmon Poetry in Ireland. She has published work in numerous journals and anthologies and is a past recipient of a Minnesota State Arts Board Fellowship in Literature. She earned her MFA from Warren Wilson College in 2004 and lives with her two teenage sons in Minneapolis.

STEPHEN MEAD's poems began appearing in literary journals in the 1990s, but after moving to Massachusetts, he concentrated on painting. In 2004 Stephen began experimenting with poetry/art hybrids, creating award-winning e-books such as "Heroines Unlikely." In 2006 he released a CD of poems set to music "Safe & Other Love Poems" as well as three DVDs. In 2007 print editions of his work were distributed online.

DENISE CALVETTI MICHAELS teaches psychology at Cascadia Community College. Her writing has been published in *Paterson Literary Review, Wetlands, Literary Mama, Bus Poems, Voices in Wartime, Milk of Almonds, Feminist Press, In Praise of Farmland,* and *Mute Note Earthward.* In 2004 she received the Crosscurrents Poetry Prize from the Washington Community College Humanities Association.

JUDITH H. MONTGOMERY's poems have received prizes from the *Bellingham Review,* the National Writers Union, *Americas Review,* and the *Red Rock Review,* as well as several Pushcart nominations. "The Photographer's Father," an honorable mention for the Randall Jarrell Poetry Award, appears in her chapbook *Passion,* which received the 2000 Oregon Book Award for Poetry. *Red Jess,* her first full-length collection, appeared in 2006 from Cherry Grove Collections; *Pulse & Constellation,* a finalist for the Finishing Line Press Chapbook Competition, appeared in June 2007.

KAY MULLEN's work has appeared in various journals, including *Valparaiso Poetry Review* and *Appalachia,* as well as the anthologies *Francis and Clare in Poetry, Washington State Poets,* and *Northwind.* She earned an MFA in creative writing from the Rainier Writing Workshop, Pacific Lutheran University. Her book *A Long Remembering: Return to Vietnam* was published by Foothills Publishers in 2006.

TIM MYERS is a writer, songwriter, storyteller, and university lecturer at Santa Clara University in Silicon Valley. He has published over one hundred poems, won a prize in a poetry contest judged by John Updike, has a poetry chapbook (*That Mass at Which the Tongue Is Celebrant,* Pecan Grove Press, 2007), won a major prize in science fiction, has been nominated for a Pushcart for an essay, and published much other fiction and nonfiction for children and adults.

DREW MYRON has been a professional writer for more than fifteen years, working as a journalist, publicist, and poet who often collaborates with artists to combine the written word with visual art. She lives on the central Oregon coast.

JIM NATAL's poetry has appeared or been reviewed in *Reed, Pool, Runes, The Paterson Literary Review,* and *Poetry International.* He has published three collections: *Talking Back to the Rocks, In the Bee Trees*—which was a finalist for the PEN Center USA Award in poetry—and *Memory and Rain,* due from Red Hen Press in 2008.

SHERYL L. NELMS was born in Marysville, Kansas. She graduated from South Dakota State University in 1979. She has had eleven books of poetry published in addition to more than 4,500 individual poems, articles, and short stories. She is the essay editor of *The Pen Woman Magazine,* a National League of American Pen Women (NLAPW) publication. She is a member of the NLAPW, the Society of Southwestern Authors, Trinity Writers Workshop, and the Abilene Writer's Guild.

PAMELA MILLER NESS is a teacher of English at the Dalton School in New York City. She has published haiku and tanka in a variety of international journals, been featured in the annual Red Moon Anthology since 1998, been anthologized in *A New Resonance II,* and published six chapbooks. Her most recent chapbook is a tanka sequence about her father's journey into Alzheimer's disease, entitled *Limbs of the Gingko* (Swamp Press, 2005).

SEAN NEVIN teaches for Arizona State University, where he is the assistant director of the Young Writer's Program and coeditor of *22 Across: A Review of Young Writers.* His poetry has appeared in *The Gettysburg Review* and the *North American Review,* among other journals. He is the recipient of a Literature Fellowship in Poetry from the National Endowment for the Arts and is the author of *A House That Falls* (Slapering Hol Press) and *Oblivio Gate* (Southern Illinois University Press), which won the Crab Orchard Award Series First Book Prize.

MAUREEN OWENS received her MFA in creative writing from Antioch University, Los Angeles, and earned her BA in literature from SUNY Binghamton. Her poetry has been anthologized in *ImageArt, Knocking on the Silence,* and *Common Intuitions.* Maureen's first book of poetry *She Sleeps With Dogs* was published by Foothills Publishing. She lives with her two greyhounds in Seneca Falls, New York.

DAVE PARSONS is recipient of an NEH Dante Fellowship (SUNY), the French/ American Legation Poetry Prize, and *descant*'s 2006 Baskerville Publishers

Poetry Prize. His first book of poems, *Editing Sky*, was winner of the Texas Review Poetry Prize and was a Violet Crown book award finalist. *Color of Mourning*, his latest collection, was released in 2007 from Texas Review Press/ Texas A&M University Press.

CANDACE PEARSON'S poetry is preoccupied with issues of memory, accountability, and the natural world. Her poems have appeared or are forthcoming in such journals as *Crab Orchard Review, Ploughshares, Runes, Rattle,* and others. She lives in the Los Angeles hills.

PAULANN PETERSEN's poetry books are *The Wild Awake* (Confluence Press), *Blood-Silk* (Quiet Lion Press), and *A Bride of Narrow Escape* (Cloudbank Books). A former Stegner Fellow at Stanford University, she serves on the board of Friends of William Stafford, organizing the January Stafford birthday events.

SCOTT PETERSON is an educator in Mattawan, Michigan. His work has appeared in *The Plains Song Review, Home and Other Places,* and *The Quarterly*. He is coauthor of *Theme Exploration: A Voyage of Discovery*. His mother passed away after a fifteen-year battle with Alzheimer's.

RONALD PIES, MD, is a physician in the department of psychiatry at Tufts University School of Medicine. He is the author of a collection of short stories (Zimmerman's Tefillin/PublishAmerica) and a book of poetry (Creeping Thyme/ Brandylane Publishers). He is also the author of *The Ethics of the Sages: An Interfaith Commentary on Pirke Avot* (Rowman & Littlefield, 2000) and *Everything Has Two Handles: A Stoic's Guide to the Art of Living* (Hamilton, 2008).

JAYNE PUPEK holds an MA in counseling psychology and has spent most of her professional life in the field of mental health. Her fiction and poetry have appeared in numerous print and online literary journals. Her poems have twice been nominated for the Pushcart Prize. She is the author of one book of poems, *Forms of Intercession* (Mayapple Press, 2008) and two chapbooks, *Local Girls* (Dead Mule, 2007) and *Primitive* (Pudding House Press, 2004). She resides near Richmond, Virginia.

ANDREW RIUTTA lives in rural Michigan with his wife, Lori, and their daughter, Issabella. His first chapbook, *The Pie in Pieces: Thirty-Three Songs from the Midwest,* was published by River Man. In 2007 he won honorable mention in the Michigan Liberal Arts Network poetry contest.

LEN ROBERTS was the author of twelve books of poetry, the most recent being *The Disappearing Trick* (University of Illinois Press, 2007). He won numerous awards for his poetry, including a Guggenheim Award, two National Endowment for the Arts Awards, and a National Endowment for the Humanities Award. A Fulbright Scholar, his book of translations *Before and After the Fall: New Poems by Sandor Csoori* was published in 2004. He died in 2007.

ELIZABETH GARTON SCANLON lives in Austin, Texas, and is the author of *A Sock Is a Pocket for Your Toes* (HarperCollins, 2004). Her poems have been published in numerous literary journals. She teaches creative writing at Austin Community College. The poem in this collection is from a series of Alzheimer's poems Scanlon wrote in honor of her grandmother, Kaye Spelletich Getz, 1918–2001.

PETER SEIDMAN was born in Chicago and was educated in the Heartland as well as on both coasts. He retired several years ago from life as a teacher, program manager, and editor to write poetry and feed hungry street folk. He lives in Berkeley, California.

JOAN I. SEIGEL's poetry has appeared in *The Atlantic Monthly, The American Scholar, Prairie Schooner,* and *The Gettysburg Review,* among other journals, and in the anthologies *Poetry Comes Up Where It Can* (University of Utah), *Blood to Remember: American Poets on the Holocaust* (Time Being Books), and *Beyond Lament* (Northwestern). Recipient of the *New Letters* Poetry Prize and the Anna Davidson Rosenberg Award, she coauthored *Peach Girl: Poems for a Chinese Daughter* (Grayson Books).

KENITH SIMMONS is professor of English and assistant vice chancellor for academic affairs at the University of Hawaii at Hilo. Her mother and father died within a month of each other in 2005, her mother of Alzheimer's and her father of vascular dementia. In addition to numerous academic articles on modern literature and film, she has published poetry in literary journals including *Paper Street, Kaimana, Malamalama, The Chaminade Literary Review, Poetica, Bridges,* and *Jewish Affairs* (South Africa).

BARBARA SIMPSON earned an MFA in creative nonfiction from Antioch University, Los Angeles. She is an Amherst Writers and Artists Affiliate and a nonfiction editor for *The Sylvan Echo.* Barbara lives in Saint Joseph, Michigan, where she is a studio artist for the Box Factory for the Arts.

BARRY SPACKS, known mainly as a poet/teacher, has also been a painter for over forty years. He teaches at University of California, Santa Barbara, was named the first poet laureate of the city of Santa Barbara in 2005, has published nine poetry collections, and has brought out three poetry-reading CDs and two novels. Over four hundred individual poems appear in paper and pixel journals. His tenth book of poems, *Food for the Journey,* was published by Cherry Grove Collections in August 2008.

CARA SPINDLER lives in Michigan and teaches high school. Her writing has appeared in *Poor Mojo's Almanac(k), Spinning Jenny,* and *Lady Churchill's Rosebud Wristlet.*

AILSA STEINERT teaches English at the Pingree School in South Hamilton, Massachusetts, and lives with her husband in nearby Manchester-By-The-Sea. She is a member of Barbara Helfgott Hyett's Workshop for Publishing Poets in Brookline, Massachusetts. Her work has appeared previously in the *Comstock Review, Orion, The Larcome Review,* and the Saltmarsh Press anthology *Rough Places Plain: Poems of the Mountains.*

MARK THALMAN's book *Catching the Limit* will be published by Bedbug Press (2008) as part of their Northwest Poetry Series. His work has appeared in *Carolina Quarterly, CutBank, Natural Bridge, Pedestal Magazine,* and *Pennsylvania Review,* among others. He received his MFA from the University of Oregon and teaches English in the public schools.

LARRY D. THOMAS has published seven collections of poems and has two additional collections in press: *The Fraternity of Oblivion* (Timberline Press, 2008) and *New and Selected Poems* (TCU Press, 2008). His poetry received the 2004 Violet Crown book award (Writers' League of Texas), 2003 Western Heritage Award (Western Heritage Museum, Oklahoma), and *Texas Review* Poetry Prizes in 2001 and 2004. In April 2007 he was appointed the 2008 Texas Poet Laureate.

GARY THOMPSON's poems have been published in a wide range of magazines, from *American Poetry Review* to *Writers' Forum;* several anthologies; and four collections, most recently *On John Muir's Trail,* from Bear Star Press, and *To the Archeologist Who Finds Us,* from Turning Point Books. He lives with his wife, Linda, on San Juan Island in Washington state.

CHRIS TUSA holds an MFA from the University of Florida. His poems have appeared in *Prairie Schooner, Texas Review, New Delta Review, The New York Quarterly, Passages North, South Dakota Review, Spoon River, The Louisville Review, Tar River Poetry, Story South, Southeast Review,* and others. Currently he teaches at Louisiana State University.

RYAN G. VAN CLEAVE's most recent books include a creative writing textbook, *Contemporary American Poetry: Behind the Scenes* (Allyn & Bacon/Longman, 2003). He teaches creative writing and literature at Clemson University.

MARTHA MODENA VERTREACE-DOODY is distinguished professor of English and poet-in-residence at Kennedy-King College, Chicago, and is a National Endowment for the Arts Fellow. Her recent work includes an essay in *In the Middle of the Middle West* (Indiana University Press) and poems anthologized in *Illinois Voices: An Anthology of Twentieth-Century Poetry* (University of Illinois Press), *Poets of the New Century* (David R. Godine Publisher), and *Manthology* (University of Iowa Press). *Glacier Fire,* her latest book, won the Word Press Poetry Prize.

DONNA WAHLERT's poetry has been published in anthologies and literary journals for over fifteen years. She has been awarded several prizes and was nominated for a Pushcart Prize. She has published a book of her poetry, *The First Pressing: Poetry of the Everyday.* The profits from her book are donated to Alzheimer's causes.

TINA WELLING writes in Jackson Hole, Wyoming. She has published essays and short fiction. Her novel *Crybaby Ranch* was published in the summer of 2008. She is a faculty member of the Jackson Hole Writers Conference.

CATHERINE WILEY was born in Rochester, New York, and has taught at the University of Colorado at Denver since 1990. Her poetry appears in *Kalliope, Salamander, Calyx, Small Pond Magazine, Copper Nickel,* a women's studies textbook, and other venues. Her chapbook *Failing Better* was a finalist for the 2004 Colorado Book Award in poetry.

MARGOT WIZANSKY's poems have appeared in a number of journals and several anthologies, including *Proposing on the Brooklyn Bridge.* In 2004 she was awarded a prize in the *Boston Herald's* Community Poetry Contest, and in 2007 in the *Northwest Cultural Council's* competition and the *American Literary Review's* competition. Also in 2007, she was a finalist in *Inkwell's* competition. She has edited two poetry anthologies, *Mercy of Tides: Poems for a Beach House* (2003) and *Rough Places Plain: Poems of the Mountains* (2006).

JEFF WORLEY's third book, *Happy Hour at the Two Keys Tavern,* won the 2007 Society of Midland Authors Literary Competition and was also named 2006 Kentucky Book of the Year in Poetry at the Southern Kentucky Book Fest. His poems have appeared in *The Threepenny Review, Poetry Northwest, The Georgia Review, New England Review, Shenandoah, The Southern Review,* and elsewhere. He works at the University of Kentucky.

GARY YOUNG's books include *Hands, The Dream of a Moral Life, Days, Braver Deeds,* winner of the Peregrine Smith Poetry Prize, and *No Other Life,* which won the William Carlos Williams Award. He has twice received fellowships from the National Endowment for the Arts, and other awards include a Pushcart Prize and a fellowship from the National Endowment for the Humanities. He edits for the Greenhouse Review Press from Santa Cruz, California.

ANDRENA ZAWINSKI was born and raised in Pittsburgh, Pennsylvania, and earned degrees at the University of Pittsburgh. She now lives and teaches writing in Oakland, California. Her full collection *Traveling in Reflected Light* was released as a Kenneth Patchen competition winner from Pig Iron Press. Her chapbook *Greatest Hits 1991–2001* is part of Pudding House's archival series. She is features editor at PoetryMagazine.com.

HOLLY ZEEB is a clinical psychologist in Watertown, Massachusetts, and has been writing poetry for thirty years. Her poems have appeared in *Snowy Egret, Pudding, Concrete Wolf, Ab Intra,* the anthologies *Fresh Water* and *Do Not Give Me Things Unbroken,* and *Tree Magic,* a CD.

MARY ZEPPA's poems have appeared in a variety of print and online journals and in several anthologies. The author of two chapbooks, *Little Ship of Blessing* (Poets Corner Press) and *The Battered Bride Overture* (Rattlesnake Press), she was a founding editor of *The Tule Review* and a coeditor (1984–95) of *Poet News.* Recipient of a 2008 Resident Fellowship from the Virginia Center for the Creative Arts, Zeppa is also one-fifth of Cherry Fizz, a quintet specializing in loose and unlabeled a cappella music.

Permissions & Acknowledgments

Arlene Ang: "Five Minutes of Silence" appeared in *Blackmail Press* 17 (2006). Reprinted by permission of the writer.

Judith Arcana: "Mamababy" was published in *Frontiers* 15.2 (1995). Reprinted by permission of the writer.

Judith Barrington: "Ineradicable" was first published in *Horses and the Human Soul* (Story Line Press, 2004). Reprinted by permission of the writer.

Marie Bahlke: "Goodwill" was published in *One Oar* (Christmas Cove Press, 2004). Reprinted by permission of the writer.

Dan Bellm: "Elegy / in advance / do not hasten" was published in the "Signals" issue of *RUNES* (2005), and in *Practice* (Sixteen Rivers Press, 2008). Reprinted by permission of the writer.

Kate Bernadette Benedict: "Recognition" was originally published in *Pierian Springs* and appeared in *Here from Away* (CustomWords, 2003). Reprinted by permission of the writer.

Bruce Berger: "Across, Down" appeared in *Facing the Music* (Confluence Press, 1995). Reprinted by permission of the writer.

Allan Douglass Coleman: "Ukiah Afternoon" was first published in *The Higginsville Reader* 7.4 (Fall 1997). "Concerning Ice Cream on Mom's Side of the Family" was first published in *Steam Ticket* 3 (1997). Both poems appear in *Like Father Like Son* (Villa Florentine Press, 2007). Reprinted by permission of the writer.

Elizabeth Cohen: "The Forgotten World" appeared in *Mother Love* (Keshet Books, 2007). Reprinted by permission of the writer.

Nina Corwin: "In Which Grandma Belle Navigates the Altoona Nursing Home" appeared in *Poetica* magazine. Reprinted by permission of the writer.

Rachel Dacus: "Elegy for an Amputation" was previously published in *Fringe* magazine. "At the Easel" appeared in *Another Circle of Delight* (Small Poetry Press, 2007). Reprinted by permission of the writer.

Nancy Dahlberg: "Confirmation" was published in *Poets Table Anthology: A Collection of Poetry by Northwest Poets* (Seattle: SCW Publications, 2002). Reprinted by permission of SCW Publications. "We All Fall Down" was published in *CALYX: A Journal of Art and Literature by Women* 19.1 (Winter 1999/2000) and in *Mute Note Earthward,* Washington Poets Association Members Anthology, vol. 1 (2004). Reprinted by permission of the writer.

Lorene Delany-Ullman: "Filler" appeared in *upstreet,* no. 3 (July 2007). Reprinted by permission of the writer.

Theodore Deppe: "Great Egrets" appeared originally in *Common Ground Review.* Reprinted by permission of the writer.

Ellen Kirvin Dudis: "Les Nuages" appeared in *The Madison Review.* "Still Life" first appeared in *Smartish Pace* and also appeared in *Off the Coast.* Reprinted by permission of the writer.

Linda Annas Ferguson: "My Mother Doesn't Know Me" also appears in *Bird Missing from One Shoulder,* © 2007 WordTech Editions, Cincinnati, Ohio.

Tess Gallagher: "She Wipes Out Time" (a slightly different version) and "Across the Border" both appeared in *Dear Ghosts,* (Graywolf Press, 2006). Copyright © 2006 by Tess Gallagher, reprinted from *Dear Ghosts,* with the permission of Graywolf Press, Saint Paul, Minnesota.

Penny Harter: "No Destination" appeared in *Along River Road* (From Here Press, 2005). Reprinted by permission of the writer.

Edward Hirsch: "Lay Back the Darkness" and "Wheeling My Father through the Alzheimer's Ward" from *Lay Back the Darkness: Poems,* copyright © 2003 by Edward Hirsch. Used by permission of Alfred A. Knopf, a division of Random House, Inc.

Kake Huck: "Death Picks Up My Aunt, Huldah Bell" was first published in *The Peralta Press* (2004). Reprinted by permission of the writer.

Holly J. Hughes: "The Bath" appeared in *Alaska Quarterly Review, Pontoon 8: An Anthology of Washington State Poets* (Floating Bridge Press, 2005) and the anthology *Family Matters: Poems of our Families* (Bottom Dog Press, 2005). Reprinted by permission of the writer.

M. J. Iuppa: "Passing the Hat" first appeared in *Tar River Poetry* and also appears in the collection *Night Traveler* (Foothills Publishing, 2003). Reprinted by permission of the writer.

Rick Kempa: "Prayer for my Mother" was published in *Passager* (2008). Reprinted by permission of the writer.

Claire Keyes: "A Little Less Than the Angels" was first published in *Currents* 5 (Portsmouth, NH: Seacoast Writers Association, 2005). Reprinted by permission of the writer.

Judy Kronenfeld: "The Withering of Their State" originally appeared in *The Women's Review of Books* 20.9 (June 2003). It was published in the chapbook *Ghost Nurseries* (Finishing Line Press, 2005) and republished in *Light Lowering in Diminished Sevenths* (Litchfield Review Press, 2008). Reprinted by permission of the writer.

Sarah Leavitt: "Kaddish" appeared in *Geist,* no. 60 (Spring 2006). Reprinted by permission of the writer.

Nancy Tupper Ling: "'The day after Auntie moves to The Maples" was previously published in *Manorborn*. Reprinted by permission of the writer.

Sybil Lockhart: "Naked" originally appeared as part of the essay "Grey" in *Literary Mama* magazine and *Literary Mama: Reading for the Maternally Inclined* (Seal Press, 2006). Reprinted by permission of the writer.

Susan Ludvigson: "Where We Have Come" was first published in *Sweet Confluence* (Louisiana State University Press, 2000). "Dreaming My Mother in the Bone Church, Kostnice" was first published in *Escaping the House of Certainty* (Louisiana State University Press, 2006). Both works are reprinted by permission of Louisiana State University Press.

David Mason: "The Inland Sea" was first published in *The Cincinnati Review* (Fall 2004). "Home Care" first appeared in *The Times Literary Supplement* (Oct. 29, 2004) and was reprinted in *Harper's* (Apr. 2005). Both are reprinted by permission of the writer.

Joel A. McCollough: "Augury" and "Returning Thanks" were published in *Poem #85*. Both poems also appeared in *Quintet* (Ninety-Six Press, Furman University, 2003). Reprinted by permission of the writer.

Ethna McKiernan: "Absences" and "Potatoes" were first published in *The One Who Swears You Can't Start Over* (Cliffs of Moher, Co. Clare, Ireland: Salmon Poetry Ltd. 2002). Reprinted by permission of Salmon Poetry.

Denise Calvetti Michaels: "Visiting Rose Haven Adult Family Home" was first published in *Wetlands Review* (2005). Reprinted by permission of the writer.

Judith H. Montgomery: "The Photographer's Father" appeared in *Passion* (Defined Providence Press, 1999). Reprinted by permission of the writer.

Drew Myron: An earlier version of "Erosion" appeared in *Central Avenue*. Reprinted by permission of the writer.

Jim Natal: "In Memory of Her Memory" is forthcoming in *Memory and Rain* (Red Hen Press, 2008). Reprinted by permission of the writer.

Sheryl Nelms: "Early Alzheimer's" appeared in *Kaleidoscope, Flimsy Excuse,* and *The Orange Willow Review*. Reprinted by permission of the writer.

Pamela Miller Ness: "A Woodpecker Taps" appeared in the chapbook *Limbs of the Gingko* (Northfield, MA: Swamp Press). Reprinted by permission of the writer.

Sean Nevin: "Losing Solomon" first appeared in JAMA: Journal *of the American Medical Association* 290.8:997 (2003). "Losing Solomon" and "Again, the Gnome and I Catch Dawn" were published in *A House That Falls* (Slapering Hol Press, 2005). Reprinted by permission of the writer.

Maureen Owens: "Carlos y Norma" appeared in *She Sleeps With Dogs* (Foothills Publishing, 2007). Reprinted by permission of the writer.

Dave Parsons: "They" was previously published in *The Texas Review* (Spring/Summer 2000) and in *Editing Sky* (Texas Review Press: Texas A&M University Press Consortium, 1999). Reprinted by permission of Texas Review Press.

Paulann Petersen: "Lane Change" was first published in *Calyx* 19.3. It appeared in *A Bride of Narrow Escape*. "Reprieve" was first published in *The Alembic* 171.4. Both appear in *A Bride of Narrow Escape* (Cloudbank Books, 2005). Reprinted by permission of the writer.

Ronald Pies: "Sonnet for a Missing Singer" was first published in *JAMA: Journal of the American Medical Association* 286 (2001): 1013. Copyright © 2001, American Medical Association. All rights reserved. Reprinted by permission of JAMA.

Jayne Pupek: "Equations" (as "Some Days" in earlier versions) appeared online in the chapbook *Local Girls* (Dead Mule, 2007) and in the collection *Forms of Intercessions* (Mayapple Press, 2008). Reprinted by permission of the writer.

Len Roberts: "My Uncle Chauncy Drove My Aunt Eleanor" from *Sweet Ones* (Minneapolis: Milkweed Editions, 1988). Copyright © 1988 by Len Roberts. Reprinted with permission from Milkweed Editions (www.milkweed.org).

Joan I. Siegel: "Letting Go" was previously published in *Yankee* (May 1996). Reprinted by permission of the writer.

Barry Spacks: "What's-Her-Name" appeared in *Regarding Women* (Cherry Grove Collections). Reprinted by permission of the writer.

Cara Spindler: The poem "Missing Script" was originally published in a five-cycle poem entitled "A Document in Madness" in *Poor Mojo's Almanac(k)*, no. 178. Reprinted by permission of the writer.

Mark Thalman: "Short-Term Memory Loss" was originally published in *Poetry Motel*. Reprinted by permission of the writer.

Larry Thomas: "Diminuendo" appeared in *JAMA: The Journal of the American Medical Association* 284.3 (2000): 280 and was also published in the collection *Where Skulls Speak Wind* (Texas Review Press, 2004). Copyright © 2000, American Medical Association. All rights reserved. Reprinted by permission of *JAMA*.

Gary Thompson: "Opera" was first published in the *Santa Clara Review* (Fall/Winter 1991). Reprinted by permission of the writer.

Donna Wahlert: "Here Let Us" was published in *Vantage Magazine* and in *The First Pressing: Poetry of the Everyday*. Reprinted by permission of the writer.

Tina Welling: "Reprieve" is included as a scene in the novel *Crybaby Ranch* (New York: NAL/Penguin, 2008). Reprinted by permission of the writer.

Jeff Worley: "His Funeral" appeared in the *Atlanta Review*. "My Father, Now on Liquids in the Tucson Nursing Home" appeared in the *Connecticut Review*. "After a Trip to the VA Hospital Alzheimer's Ward, Tucson" appeared in the *Florida Review*. "His Funeral" won the *Atlanta Review*'s 2002 International Poetry Competition Grand Prize. All are reprinted by permission of the writer.

Gary Young: "Rev. Robert A. Young" first appeared in *Hands* (Jazz Press, 1981). Reprinted by permission of the writer.

Andrena Zawinski: "Hot Flashes" was published in the *Onion River Review* 3.1 (Goddard College). Reprinted by permission of the writer.